TEETH WHITENING AT HOME
THE 6 BEST PRODUCTS EXPLORED AND COMPARED

written in collaboration with seven
distinguished dental experts

George Ghidrai
MD

Copyright © 2024 George Ghidrai
All rights reserved.
ISBN: 979-834-69-5328-9

Contents

1. Introduction — pg. 1
2. General Considerations — pg. 6
2.1 Causes of staining and tooth discoloration — pg. 7
2.2 Types of staining — pg. 9
2.3 Teeth whitening products and methods — pg. 10
2.4 How to make teeth whitening last longer — pg. 12
3. Comparing all teeth whitening products — pg. 16
4. Teeth whitening strips — pg. 23
5. Teeth whitening trays and gel — pg. 34
6. LED Teeth Whitening — pg. 46
7. Teeth Whitening Pens — pg. 55
8. Teeth whitening toothpaste — pg. 64
9. Teeth whitening rinses — pg. 74
10. Conclusions — pg. 82
Our experts — pg. 86

References — pg. 92
About The Author — pg. 94

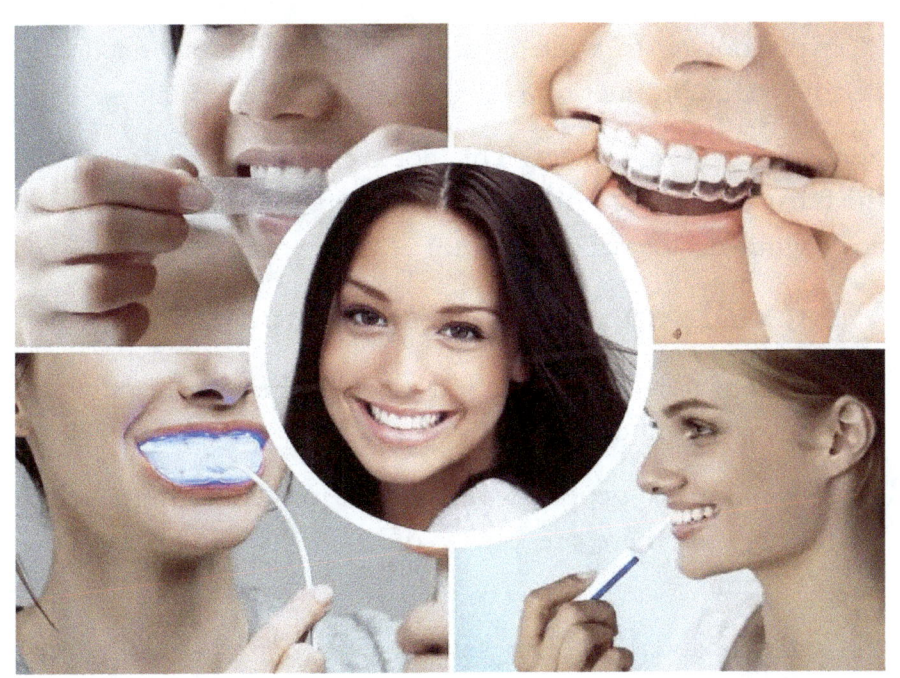

1. Introduction

Are you looking to whiten your teeth at home but need help deciding what product to use?

You are in the right place. This book **explores and compares** the most efficient at-home teeth whitening products so you can confidently decide which ones are best for your needs.

What will you learn from this book?

This book is not just a guide but a comprehensive resource on at-home teeth whitening.

Today, countless people worldwide resort to at-home teeth whitening, and there are plenty of products and methods to choose from.

You may be able to whiten your teeth at home naturally using products you can find in the grocery store, following a diet rich in fruits and vegetables, or making specific lifestyle changes.

However, this book **will mainly concentrate on 6 types of at-home teeth whitening products that have proved most effective in our days**. You can safely use natural remedies alongside these products if you wish.

These are the 6 products that we will discuss and compare throughout our book. They are widely used nowadays, and many of you have probably tried them or are planning to do so.

- Whitening strips
- Whitening gels
- LED light whitening
- Whitening pens

TEETH WHITENING AT HOME
THE 6 BEST PRODUCTS EXPLORED AND COMPARED

- Whitening toothpaste
- Whitening mouthwashes

We will start with some general considerations, discussing the causes of staining and tooth discoloration and the types of stains that can develop on your teeth. You will then learn how teeth whitening works and how to keep your teeth white for longer.

You will find a comparison table with key features of all teeth whitening methods, helping you quickly determine which is best for your needs.

We will then dive into the central part of our book that evaluates and explores each type of whitening product. To get most of your read, we will answer 8 key questions:

1. How does the procedure work?
2. What to expect from the product?
3. How long does it take to work?
4. What should you look for when purchasing these types of products?
5. What are the pros and benefits?
6. What are the risks and drawbacks?
7. How to use the product?
8. How long does a treatment with this procedure last?

By comparing the answers for each type of product, you will be able to understand:

- What whitening procedures work best and why

- What are the safest products, and which can occasionally cause side effects

- When should you use each method, and why it's sometimes important to rely on more than one whitening procedure

- What is the best whitening "plan" for you

- Critical features for each method

- And many more

At the end of each chapter, we recommend two of the best products available based on our dental expert's experience and expertise.

Our recommendations don't imply that you will get the best results only when using these products. Other products on the market can also be highly efficient.

It is just that the products we recommend have been studied (and tested) by our experts on many patients, and the final results were excellent.

Our dental experts

This book was written in collaboration with 7 distinguished dental experts.

Our experts are not just dental professionals but well-established figures with rich experience and expertise in cosmetic dentistry. They have recommended and supervised at-home teeth whitening procedures for thousands of patients, making their opinion on the subject invaluable.

Our dental experts gave us valuable insights, and their knowledge and expertise are highlighted throughout the book.

You can find the list of our experts and their credentials at the end of the book.

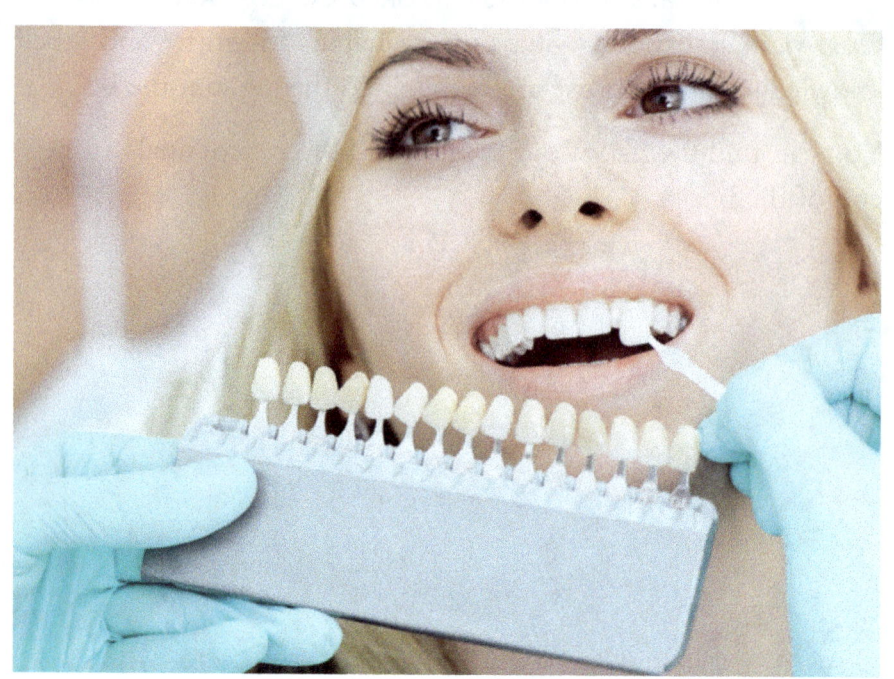

2. General considerations

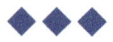

First, we will discuss some general aspects of tooth staining and discoloration, and fundamental points about teeth whitening procedures and products.

2.1 Causes of staining and tooth discoloration

These are the most significant factors that can stain or discolor your teeth:

Staining foods and drinks

A high intake of foods and drinks, such as coffee, red wine, tea, colas, and various fruits or vegetables (berries, apples, potatoes, etc.) can stain your teeth over time.

Smoking or the use of tobacco products

Research indicates that tooth discoloration is more common among people who smoke compared to people who don't. Moreover, heavy smokers tend to have yellow or, more frequently, brown teeth.

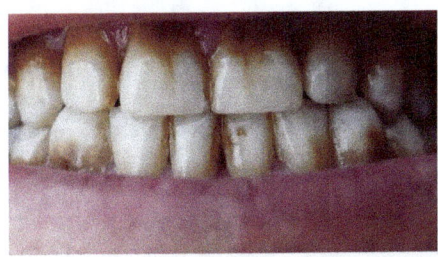
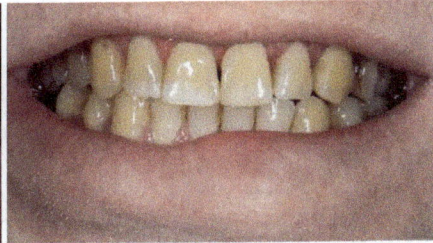

teeth stains caused by smoking   *teeth stains caused by coffee*

Poor dental hygiene

If plaque is not removed with regular brushing and flossing, you're more likely to develop discolored teeth.

Medications

Medications such as allergy and blood pressure drugs, or certain antibiotics (like tetracycline) can cause teeth stains or a reduction in the brilliance of the enamel.

Diseases

Several general health conditions, including liver disease, calcium deficiency, eating disorders, and metabolic diseases, can cause teeth discoloration.

Moreover, treatments for some conditions can also affect tooth color. For example, head and neck radiation and chemotherapy can cause teeth discoloration. In addition, certain infections in pregnant mothers can lead to tooth discoloration in their babies by affecting enamel development.

Dental trauma

Falls and sports-related injuries can cause trauma that results in tooth discoloration.

Tooth decay

Tooth decay will also change the appearance of your teeth, resulting in black or brown spots.

Aging

As a person ages, adult teeth often become darker due to changes in their mineral structure.

Different color meanings

In many cases, the color of your teeth or the stains that form on your teeth can pinpoint the cause.

- **Yellow** stains are usually caused by eating and drinking dark-colored foods or beverages. They may also mean that you need to improve your oral hygiene.

- **Brown** teeth discoloration is a result of smoking or chewing tobacco products. Brown stains may also indicate tooth cavities.

- **Gray** tooth discoloration may mean the nerve inside your tooth is severely affected. Dental trauma or a dental cavity that has reached the pulp can cause this.

- **Black** spots on your teeth typically indicate areas of severe decay.

Scott Cardall, DMD, MS, Owner Orthodontist at Orem Orthodontics, states: "Bleaching is less effective on grayish-tinted teeth, while it sometimes improves brown teeth. Yellowish teeth, on the other hand, tend to respond best."

On the other hand, treating your cavities, improving your oral hygiene, and quitting smoking are also essential steps in the whitening process.

2.2 Types of staining

Two types of stains can develop on teeth. Each has different origins and requires different types of whitening procedures.

a. Extrinsic stains

Extrinsic stains (or external stains) originate from external sources, such as drinks, foods, or tobacco. External stains remain on the tooth's surface and do not soak into the tooth structure beneath.

As a result, these stains are easier to deal with, and most over-the-counter whitening products may help lessen their appearance.

b. Intrinsic stains

Intrinsic stains (or internal stains) generally start inside the tooth; aging and internal decay are two examples of intrinsic stains. Other types of internal stains may also come from color pigments found in food and beverages and habits like smoking. These stains penetrate more deeply into the teeth and can cause a yellowish color.

Stronger bleaching products from professional whitening are required to correct intrinsic stains.

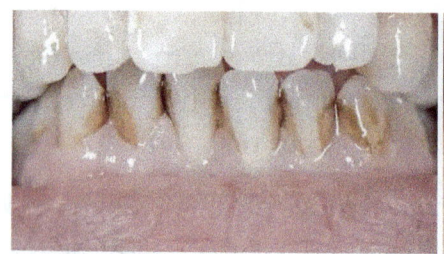

extrinsic stains

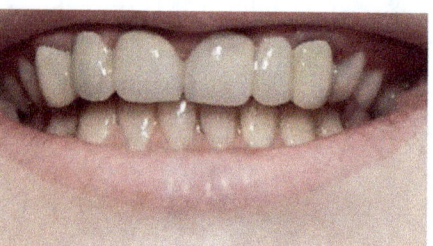

intrinsic stains:
teeth discoloration caused by aging

2.3 Teeth whitening products and methods

A person can get whitening products or services:

1. **Through their dentist**: Dentist-supplied whitening products are more concentrated and thus more effective than over-the-counter products.

Professional teeth whitening is performed at the dental office. The process involves applying whitening gel to your teeth. A heating lamp, zoom light, or laser is aimed at the teeth for 20-minute intervals.

Dentists can also supply patients with professional whitening strips, gels, or rinses. These are more concentrated than similar over-the-counter products.

2. **Over-the-counter products** include whitening strips, gels, whitening pens, whitening toothpaste, and rinses. We will discuss and compare all these products throughout our book.

How does teeth whitening work?

All teeth whitening products contain a *bleaching agent*. This can be either hydrogen peroxide or carbamide peroxide. There is no significant difference in the effectiveness of the two bleaching agents.

Generally, at-home teeth whitening products contain a lower concentration of active ingredients than professional in-office teeth whitening methods.

For example, in-office whitening gels contain 25% to 40% hydrogen peroxide, over-the-counter gels around 10%, and whitening rinses only 2%.

When left in contact with your teeth, the bleaching agent breaks the stains into smaller pieces. This will make the stains less concentrated, and the visual appearance of your teeth will look brighter.

The amount of active ingredient determines the effectiveness of the whitening process. Although at-home bleaching products work, they may not produce results equal to those of in-office bleaching procedures.

Important tips before you start a teeth whitening treatment

- It is crucial to discuss the use of these products with a dentist.

- Teeth whitening products do not work on fake teeth, such as crowns, veneers or fillings.

- You should carefully read any information on the product's packaging and instructions before using any at-home teeth whitening methods.

- If you are aware of any ongoing dental conditions, such as gum disease or teeth sensitivity, you should consult your dentist before using any at-home teeth whitening products.

2.4 How to make the teeth whitening process last longer

There are several steps you can take to make the results of the teeth whitening procedure last longer:

- **Regular and proper oral hygiene**

Good oral hygiene habits are essential for keeping teeth and gums healthy and maintaining their whiteness for longer.

This means brushing your teeth at least twice daily, flossing to reduce plaque in hard-to-reach places, and rinsing the mouth with an antiseptic mouthwash to reduce plaque-causing bacteria.

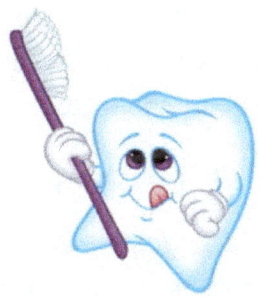

- **Avoid staining foods or drinks**

Try to reduce your intake of staining foods and drinks such as coffee, tea, red wine, blueberries, and colored beverages. If not drinking beverages seems too challenging, you may use a straw to limit how much of the pigmented drink touches the whitened teeth.

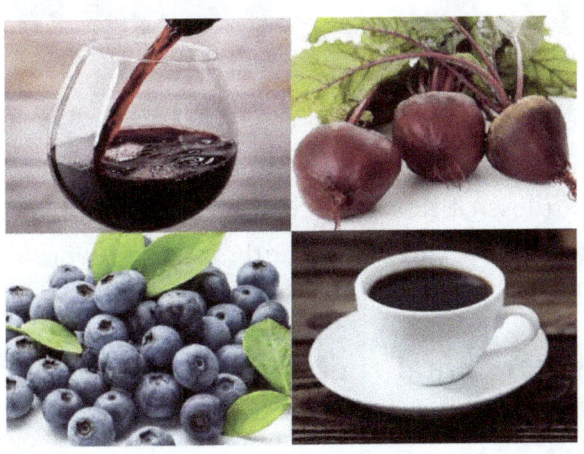

- **Rinse with water**

    Sometimes, avoiding all kinds of staining foods may be difficult. After all, you do want to drink your cup of coffee in the morning, eat your blueberries, or have a glass of red wine. If this is the case, rinse with plenty of water just after the intake to reduce the staining.

- **Quit smoking or tobacco products**

Unfortunately, when it comes to smoking and tobacco products, the only practical approach is quitting them altogether.

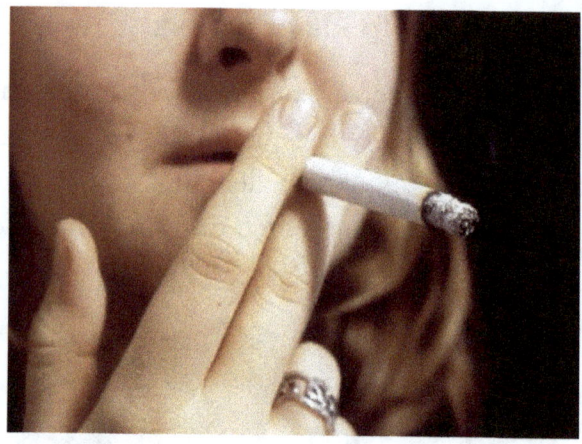

Regardless of how long you have used tobacco products, quitting now can significantly reduce severe risks to your health, and it will also keep your teeth white for longer.

- **Regular dental checkups**

    Dental appointments for checkups and cleanings are essential. The dentist will polish your teeth, remove the hardened plaque (called calculus or tartar), and deal with the stubborn stains. Ideally, this should happen every six months to keep the smile in good shape.

- **Combine teeth whitening products**

Most of the time, you will have to use more than a single product for optimum results.

For example, after a professional teeth whitening procedure, your dentist may recommend you use a whitening toothpaste to reduce surface stains. Rinsing regularly with whitening mouthwashes may be another effective option.

	PRODUCT	PRODUCT	PRODUCT
Feature 1	✓	✓	✓
Feature 2	✓	✓	✗
Feature 3	✓	✓	✓
Feature 4	✗	✓	✓

3. Comparing all teeth whitening products

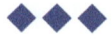

On the following pages, you can find 4 comparison tables with the key features of all teeth whitening methods (including professional, in-office whitening) set side by side.

Here, you can compare all the methods at a glance to quickly determine which might be best for your needs.

	Teeth whitening strips	Whitening trays over-the-counter
Whitening effectiveness	moderate	moderate to high
Main indications	mild discoloration, minor staining	mild to moderate staining or discoloration
Ease of use	easy to use	moderate
Side effects probability	high	moderate to high
Price	medium	medium to high
Observations	• not advisable if you have sensitive teeth	• the tray fit is not as comfortable as with custom-made trays • bleaching gel contains less amount of active ingredients

TEETH WHITENING AT HOME
THE 6 BEST PRODUCTS EXPLORED AND COMPARED

	Whitening trays custom-made	LED Teeth Whitening
Whitening effectiveness	high	moderate to high
Main indications	moderate to high staining or discoloration	moderate to high staining or discoloration
Ease of use	moderate	moderate
Side effects probability	low	moderate to high
Price	high	high
Observations	• side effects are minimal because the custom tray fits perfectly • bleaching gel contains more active ingredients	• the whitening is the result of the gel and only partly of the LED light • possible side effects if the LED light is misused

	Teeth Whitening Pens	Teeth whitening toothpaste
Whitening effectiveness	low to moderate	very low
Main indications	minor touch-ups to your teeth's whiteness	prevent and reduce external stains
Ease of use	very easy to use	very easy to use
Side effects probability	low to moderate	very low
Price	low	very low
Observations	• best used as a maintenance option between other whitening treatments	• a way to maintain teeth's brightness and prolong professional treatment results • designed for regular, long-term use

TEETH WHITENING AT HOME
THE 6 BEST PRODUCTS EXPLORED AND COMPARED

	Teeth whitening rinses	Professional teeth whitening
Whitening effectiveness	low	very high
Main indications	removing surface stains	all types of staining and discoloration
Ease of use	easy to use	in-office procedure
Side effects probability	low	moderate
Price	low	very high
Observations	• best used in combination with other methods • designed for long-term use	• the procedure is supervised to limit side-effects • considered the most effective whitening method

In the coming chapters, we will detail all at-home teeth whitening methods and explain everything you need to know.

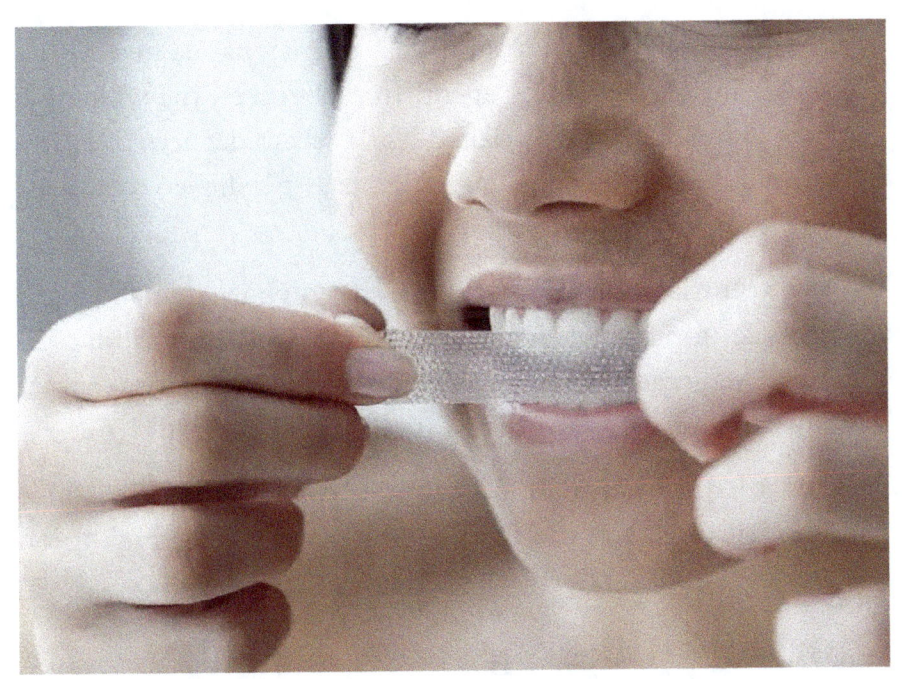

4. Teeth whitening strips

◆◆◆

Teeth whitening strips are thin layers of material coated with a gel containing the bleaching agent. In most cases, the whitening agent is either hydrogen peroxide or carbamide peroxide, but other ingredients, such as baking soda, specific enzymes, or chlorine dioxide, can be used.

Usually, you will apply the strips directly to your teeth and leave them there for the recommended time (generally about 30 minutes). Manufacturers will also suggest the ideal frequency of use and the total length of the treatment.

A standard recommendation is to apply whitening strips once daily for 14 days, but the instructions may vary depending on the product.

How do whitening strips work?

When you wear the strips over your teeth, the active bleaching gel comes into contact with them. In most cases, the whitening agent is peroxide (hydrogen peroxide or carbamide peroxide), an ingredient used in many professional whitening treatments.

Peroxides will penetrate the enamel and enter the deeper dentin layer. Here, they will act by breaking down the pigments that cause staining. As a result, these agents can lighten your teeth by a shade or two.

Some whitening strips contain baking soda or enzymes as active ingredients. They are usually gentler on the teeth, but the whitening effects will not be as visible and long-lasting.

What to expect from whitening strips?

It is essential to set your goals before you begin the treatment and not have unrealistic expectations.

Whitening strips are proven to work if correctly used, but the results are less noticeable than with professional whitening.

Scott Cardall, DMD, MS, Owner Orthodontist at Orem Orthodontics, expects whitening strips to work, especially with patients who haven't whitened their teeth in the past.

Whitening strips work best in the case of:

- mild discoloration
- minor staining
- stains from lifestyle habits like drinking coffee or smoking
- they can also be a good option for keeping your teeth white after having pro whitening done

Whitening strips may not give you the desired results in the following situations:

- heavy staining
- stains occurring from plaque and tartar build-up
- health issues or reactions to medication
- whitening strips may also create discomfort if you have sensitive teeth

In later cases, you should visit your dentist for an in-office bleaching session and to address the source of the stains.

Dr. Zev Schulhof, Iconic Implants, would not recommend the whitening strips for all his patients. "Those with significant staining and discoloration, for instance, will get better results from professional treatments. However, for those with very mild discoloration and no sensitivity, these strips can provide noticeable results within a week or two", says Dr. Zev Schulhof.

How long do whitening strips take to work?

Sometimes, you may see the first results in as little as 3 to 4 days, but it is more common that the first noticeable results appear after you use the strips for a minimum of 7 days.

This largely depends on the level of staining and the product you use. More advanced whitening strips claim results as early as 3 days, but it is still being determined if they will deliver.

From Jerry Friedman, DDS experience: "If you have mild to moderate surface stains, whitening strips can help you achieve noticeable whiter teeth in just a couple of weeks."

What should you look for when purchasing teeth whitening strips?

If you are planning to use teeth whitening strips, there are several things to consider when shopping for the product:

Ingredients

Whitening strips that contain hydrogen peroxide or carbamide peroxide as active ingredients have better whitening results. Moreover, the amount of active ingredients in the whitening strips determines their effectiveness at whitening your teeth.

Peroxide-based strips typically contain between 10% and 22% hydrogen peroxide or 3% to 15% carbamide peroxide, depending on the brand.

You may discuss these issues with your dentist, as selecting the strip with the highest amount of bleaching agent is not always advisable. Products with a high percentage of active ingredients will have better bleaching results. However, you will also be at a higher risk of developing side effects such as teeth sensitivity or gum irritation, especially in case of ongoing mouth conditions.

Jasveen Singh, DMD, Pediatric Dentist and the Owner of Pediatric Dentistry And Beyond in Boston, stresses the importance of talking with your dentist before you start using the strips: "This step will make sure that you pick a product that's best suited for your dental health and that you're using it correctly. Remember, the goal is a brighter smile without compromising your teeth and gums!."

Make sure the product does not contain other ingredients that could damage your teeth or gums.

Dental organizations approval

Products with the ADA Seal of Acceptance or approvals from other dental organizations should be safer.

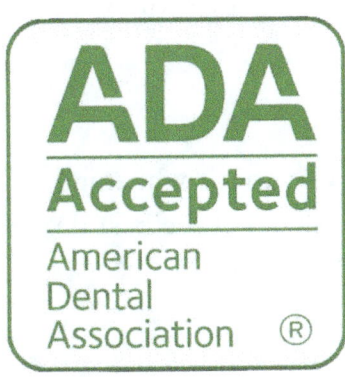

Read the instructions

Check out the promised results so you can compare them to other products.

If you have sensitive teeth

If you have sensitive teeth, it is advisable to opt for another whitening method, as Dr. Jerry Friedman, North Jersey Oral & Maxillofacial Surgery, suggests:

"I wouldn't suggest them for patients with sensitive teeth because the ingredients in whitening strips can cause discomfort for these individuals."

Customer reviews

If you read the product's online reviews, you can find answers to many questions:

- how effective is the product?
- does the treatment create any discomfort?
- how long does the treatment take?
- how effective is it in the long term?

Keep in mind, though, that the outcome may be different for every patient, and what works for one patient might not work for another.

Price

Compare the prices of various whitening strips at the same time with their effectiveness to get the best deal possible.

Teeth whitening strips pros

The benefits of using whitening strips may include:

- easy to use from the comfort of your home
- affordable price, particularly compared to professional procedures
- you generally get good results if you use them correctly, mainly in case of mild discoloration or minor staining
- simple to obtain without needing to visit your dentist

Jasveen Singh, DMD: "I usually recommend these strips to those eager to brighten their smiles from the comfort of their home. They're not only affordable but pretty simple to use."

Risks and drawbacks

Although they have many advantages, there are also some downsides and risks you need to be aware of.

- The strips can cause side effects, such as teeth sensitivity or gum irritation. These side effects are more likely to occur:
  - in case of the overuse of these products
  - when you do not use the whitening strips as specified in the product's instructions
  - in case of ongoing mouth conditions, such as gum disease or tooth sensitivity

Shahrooz Yazdani, DDS, CEO and Director of Yazdani Family Dentistry and Costello Family Dentistry, recommends using toothpaste formulated for sensitive

- teeth in such cases to help rebuild the protective layer of your teeth.

- The overuse of these products can also damage your teeth.

- Sometimes, it can be challenging to keep the strips in place.

- Some patients will need to take several sessions to get the desired results.

- Whitening strips do not give the desired outcome in case of severe staining, and the bleaching effects are not as dramatic as those of professional whitening. Consequently, patients with high expectations might be disappointed by the results.

How to use whitening strips?

Please read the instructions and any additional information carefully. You should use the product as recommended. Keep in mind that each type of whitening strip may have different instructions.

1. Brush your teeth

Brush and floss your teeth, then wait at least 30 minutes before applying the strips. Some specialists will instruct you not to use fluoride toothpaste before using the strips, as fluoride could interfere with the bleaching agent. If this is the case, use a non-fluoride toothpaste or brush without toothpaste.

2. Apply the strips

Typically, you will apply the whitening strips directly over your teeth. Peel the strip and use it along the gums. You need to apply strips to both your upper and lower teeth.

3. Wait for the recommended time

In most cases, you will leave the strips on for 30 minutes twice daily for two weeks. However, these may differ depending on the product.

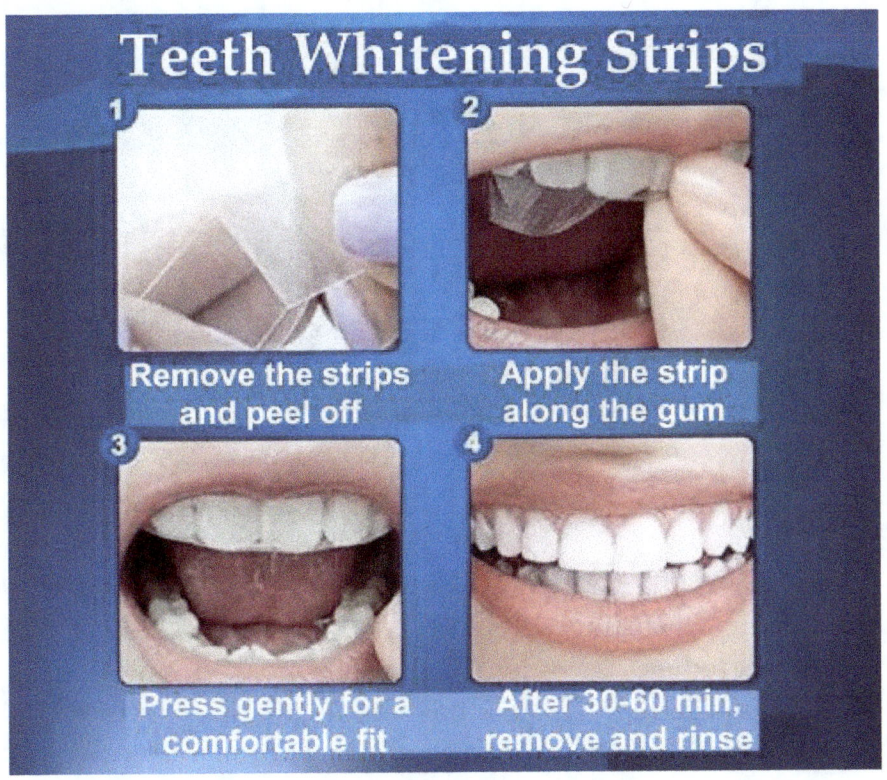

How long does a treatment with whitening strips last?

A treatment with whitening strips can last up to 6 months. To maximize the effect, follow the tips for keeping your teeth white (see subchapter 2.4).

Best products: Whitening Strips

- **Crest 3D Whitestrips Professional Effects**

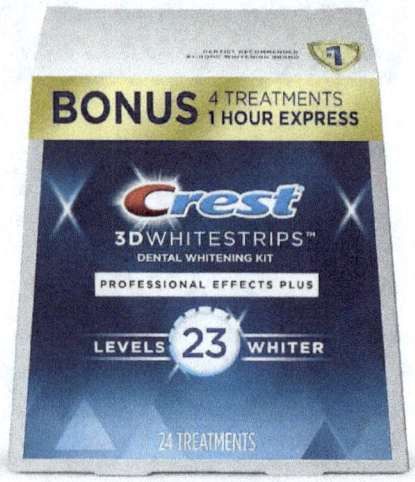

Scott Cardall, DMD, MS: "Crest 3D Whitestrips Professional Effects with 10% hydrogen peroxide as the active ingredient is one of the better whitening strips available in 2024. It also has many positive reviews on Amazon and other eCommerce sites."

- Oral-B 3D White Whitestrips

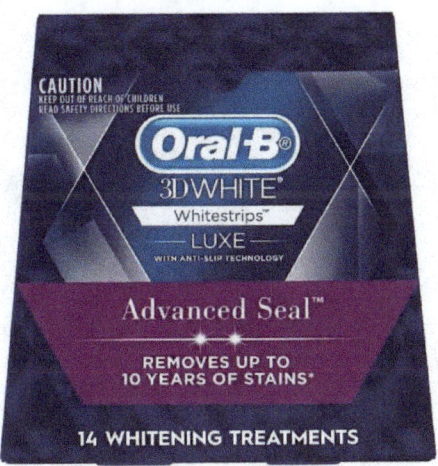

Jasveen Singh, DMD: "I've been recommending Oral-B 3D White Whitestrips to people looking for an easy way to brighten their smiles at home. They really stick tightly to your teeth, so you even get a whitening across your whole smile. Plus, they're with hydrogen peroxide, which is great for busting stains. Most people I talk to find that they feel less sensitivity with these compared to other brands."

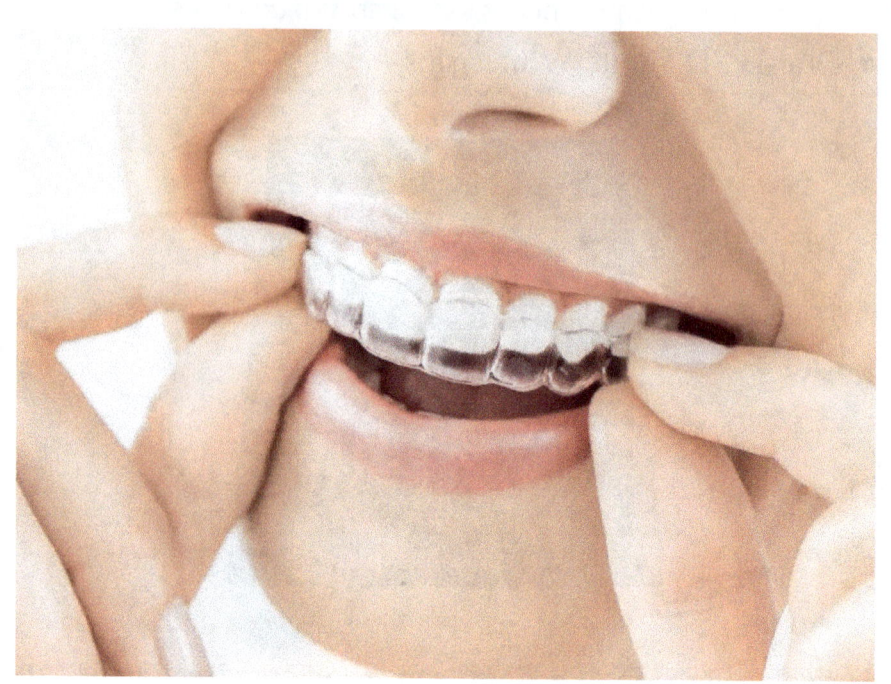

5. Teeth whitening trays and gel

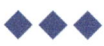

Teeth whitening treatments with whitening trays involve using a tooth tray and bleaching gel inserted into the tooth tray to activate the whitening process.

Two types of trays may be used during this process:

1. **Over-the-counter teeth whitening trays** are typically made of a flexible material that molds to your teeth.

2. **Custom-made trays** are created in-office by your dentist to perfectly fit your teeth. Although more expensive, they offer a superior fit compared to over-the-counter trays.

A teeth whitening treatment with whitening trays typically takes 15 days to a month. You apply the whitening trays to your teeth for at least 4 hours every day. Sometimes, you will be advised to wear the trays the entire night.

How do teeth whitening trays work?

The whitening gel inserted in the trays contains either hydrogen peroxide or carbamide peroxide as active ingredients.

When left in contact with your teeth, the bleaching agents will penetrate through the enamel (which is transparent) and reach the dentin, the underlying structure that gives teeth their color.

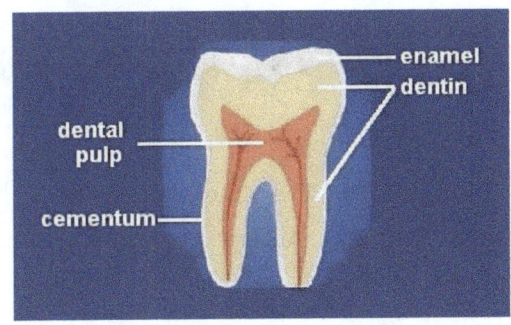

As the gel remains fixed on your teeth for a prolonged time, the peroxides will act on the stains by breaking them down, carrying out their work for hours.

What to expect from whitening trays?

Whitening trays are designed to stay on your teeth for a more extended period. Compared to whitening strips, usually held for around 30 minutes, teeth-whitening trays should remain on your teeth for at least 4 hours.

Whitening trays are not intended to work fast. Instead, you will notice a gradual whitening of your teeth. This type of teeth whitening has two crucial advantages:

- The effects of dental sensitivity are minimized, and the enamel is fully protected while the dentin is whitened. It is considered one of the safest methods of teeth whitening.

- Thanks to the constant whitening process, it is possible to lighten several shades of the color of the teeth, sometimes achieving dramatic changes.

Dr. Jerry Friedman, North Jersey Oral & Maxillofacial Surgery, is positive that at-home whitening gels can provide surprisingly great results.

How long do whitening trays take to work?

It may take 7 to 14 days to notice the first results. However, when they do appear, the changes can be significant, with minimal side effects.

What should you look for when you plan to whiten your teeth with whitening trays?

The key aspect is deciding between an over-the-counter product and one supplied by your dentist to use at home.

- **Over-the-counter teeth whitening tray system**

Over-the-counter teeth whitening trays are typically made of a flexible material that molds to your teeth. Some teeth whitening trays are prefilled with a peroxide-based whitening agent, while others come with syringes of whitening gel.

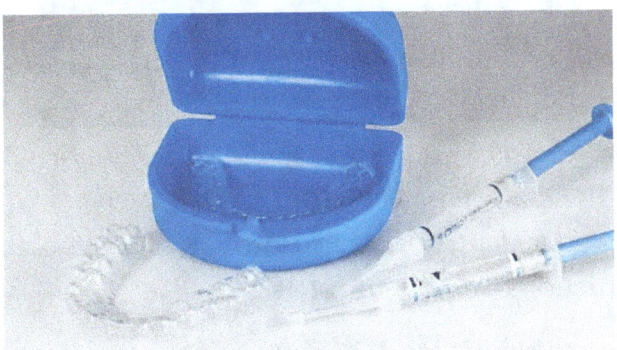

over-the-counter teeth whitening tray system

Many systems will include a complete set of disposable trays; you use two trays per day, one for your bottom teeth and one for your top teeth.

While over-the-counter teeth whitening trays and bleaching products are much cheaper, there are many benefits to opting for professional custom-made trays.

- **Teeth whitening tray system supplied by the dentist**

In this scenario, the trays are custom-made to fit your mouth perfectly. The dentist takes an impression of your two dental arches, and the dental laboratory will manufacture two custom trays to fit your upper and lower teeth.

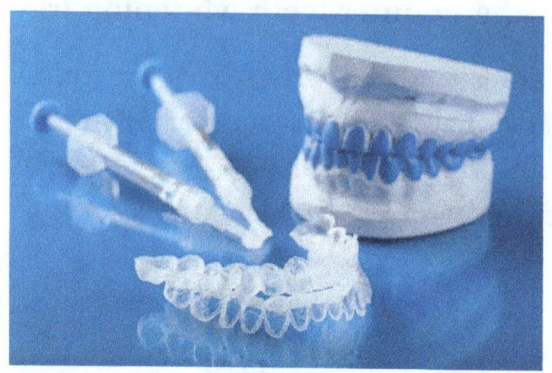

teeth whitening tray system supplied by the dentist; the trays are manufactured on the dental mold

Moreover, your dentist may also provide the bleaching gel and exact instructions on how to use it.

In-office teeth whitening tray systems are more expensive, but they also come with significant advantages:

○ The custom trays will give you a comfortable fit. Because they perfectly fit your teeth, they also prevent the gel from leaking and irritating the gum tissue.

○ The whitening gel usually contains a higher amount of active ingredients, making the whitening process more effective.

Shahrooz Yazdani, DDS, CEO and Director of Yazdani Family Dentistry and Costello Family Dentistry, believes custom-made trays with dentist-provided bleaching gel are one of the most effective at-home teeth whitening methods:

"We recommend dentist-provided whitening kits. They save patients time and money as they are more effective and personalized than drugstore products and don't require patients to come into the office for multiple treatments. We like to use at-home kits, which involve using custom trays that you wear over your teeth each day to achieve results over a more extended period," Dr. Yazdani says.

Teeth whitening trays pros

- It is one of the most effective at-home teeth whitening procedures. If carried out correctly, it can lighten several shades of tooth color.

- The effects of tooth sensitivity and gum irritation are minimized, particularly if you use custom-made trays.

- Affordable price compared to professional methods. Although more expensive than whitening strips, whitening trays are cheaper than professional, in-office treatments. Keep in mind that custom tray systems are more expensive than over-the-counter products.

"At-home custom-tray whitening is less expensive than in-office whitening treatments but can achieve the same results with patients who use them as directed," Scott Cardall, DMD, MS, points out.

Risks and drawbacks

Side effects generally occur when products are overused or when patients do not follow the exact recommendations.

Even with custom-made trays, some patients can experience increased tooth sensitivity. However, after the treatment stops, tooth sensitivity will gradually disappear, and the teeth will return to their normal state.

In such cases, the dentist may recommend a break in the treatment. This way, the therapy with whitening trays can be extended to one month or even more.

When over-the-counter trays are used, the risk of developing side effects such as gum irritation is higher. That's because these trays are not designed to fit every size of dental arch.

Scott Cardall, DMD, MS, Owner Orthodontist at Orem Orthodontics, is convinced that "**compared to one-size-fits-all trays that may run large and loose, custom whitening trays are custom-crafted to fit snugly around your unique teeth. These trays also prevent gum irritation as they keep the gel from leaking out onto the gum tissue.**"

How to use whitening trays?

If you decide to use custom-made trays, the first step is to visit your dentist, who will manufacture the trays. If you use over-the-counter trays, the whitening kit will supply both the flexible trays and the bleaching gel.

Dr. Scott Cardall recommends custom-fitted whitening trays with professional-grade whitening gels for home use. He believes these trays ensure better contact between the whitening agent and teeth, leading to more consistent whitening results while also preventing gum irritation.

Here is the process step-by-step:

1. Dental impressions

Your dentist will take impressions of your teeth and use them to create dental molds for your upper and lower teeth.

2. Custom-made trays manufacture

The dental lab will then manufacture two custom-made trays, one for your upper and one for your lower teeth. The dentist will give you the trays and precise instructions on how to use them. In many cases, your dentist will also supply the whitening gel or indicate where you should purchase it.

3. Brushing your teeth

Brush and floss your teeth before using the whitening trays. Wait for at least 30 minutes before applying the trays to your teeth.

4. Inserting the whitening gel

Insert the whitening gel in the tooth trays. It is essential to apply the exact amount recommended in the instructions.

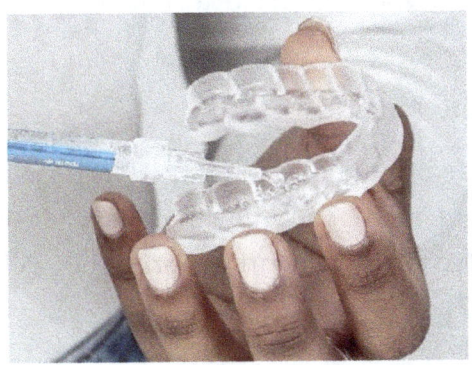

Sometimes, when you use over-the-counter systems, the trays can be prefilled with the exact quantity of bleaching agent.

5. Putting on the trays

Push the trays firmly into place against your teeth. Use a cloth to wipe off any gel that leaks out from the trays to prevent gum irritation.

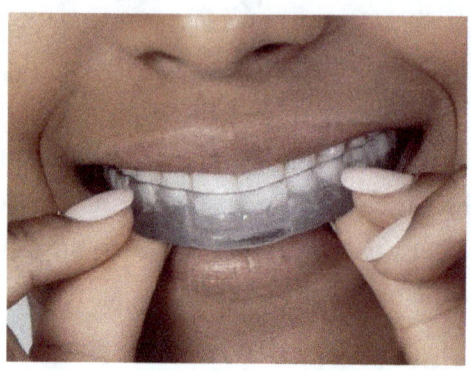

6. Wear the trays as instructed

It is imperative to wear the trays precisely as recommended. Some bleaching gels should be held in place for 4 hours, while others will be worn the entire night.

Generally, bleaching gels with more peroxide are worn for shorter amounts of time. If any burning or increased tooth sensitivity occurs, you may need to take off the trays early and inform your doctor.

7. Cleaning the solution

When the time is up, remove the trays and rinse the teeth. Use a toothbrush to remove any remaining gel. If you experience tooth sensitivity, a desensitizing toothpaste will help improve the situation.

8. Clean and store the trays

Clean and wipe all the gel off the trays before placing them in a holder until the next use. Store the syringe with the remaining gel in a cold place.

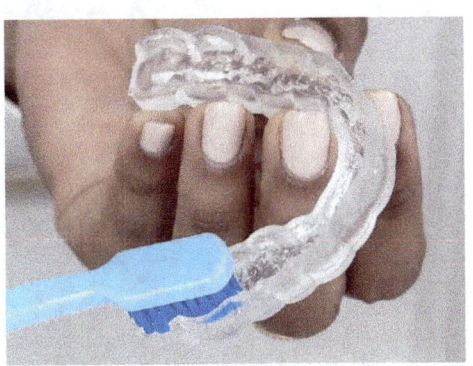

How long does a treatment with whitening trays last?

A treatment with whitening trays will last 6 months or even up to one year if you practice good maintenance measures.

This means:

- brushing your teeth, flossing, and rinsing the mouth with an antiseptic mouthwash
- reducing the intake of staining foods and drinks
- rinsing with water after the intake of staining foods
- quitting smoking or tobacco products
- regular dental checkups

Best products: Whitening Trays and Gel

- Custom-made trays with professional whitening gel

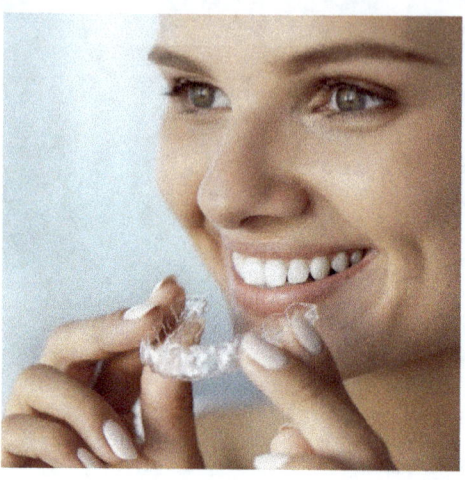

Most experts recommend custom whitening trays with professional gel as the best at-home teeth whitening option.

Scott Cardall, DMD, MS: "I recommend custom-fitted whitening trays with professional-grade whitening gels to be worn at home. This ensures better contact between the whitening agent and teeth, leading to more consistent whitening results."

To use custom-made trays, you must visit your dentist, who will manufacture the trays, provide the whitening gel, and give you precise instructions on how to use it.

- **Opalescence Go Prefilled Whitening Trays**

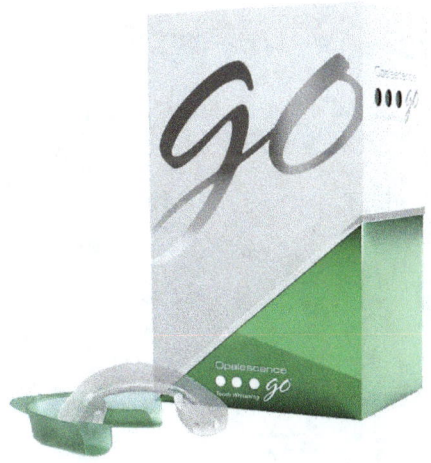

George Ghidrai, MD: "Opalescence Go Trays are very easy to use as each tray is prefilled with the required quantity of gel. The results were very encouraging from my experience with patients who used this formula. The tray fit is relatively comfortable, although it can't match custom-made trays."

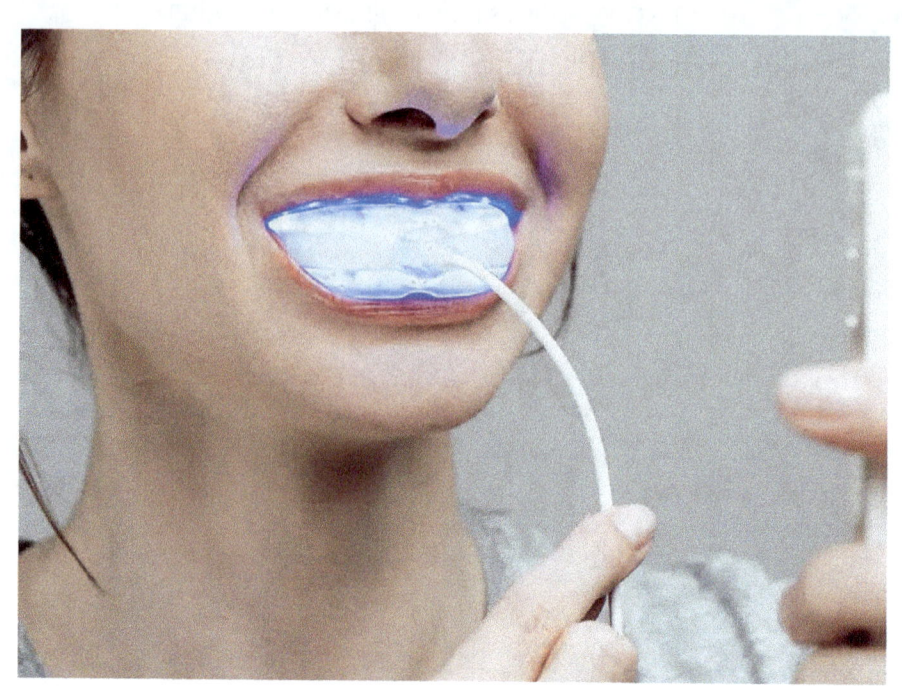

6. LED Teeth Whitening

LED whitening is a process in which an LED light is used in combination with a whitening gel.

There are two types of LED Teeth Whitening:

- in-office LED Teeth Whitening
- at-home LED Teeth Whitening kits

How does LED teeth whitening work?

LED teeth whitening uses the same types of gels as teeth whitening trays. The only difference is the LED device that claims to accelerate the process.

The exposure of the whitening gel to the LED light helps activate the process. It causes the gel to break up and start a chemical reaction that will lift the stains from your teeth.

What to expect from LED teeth whitening?

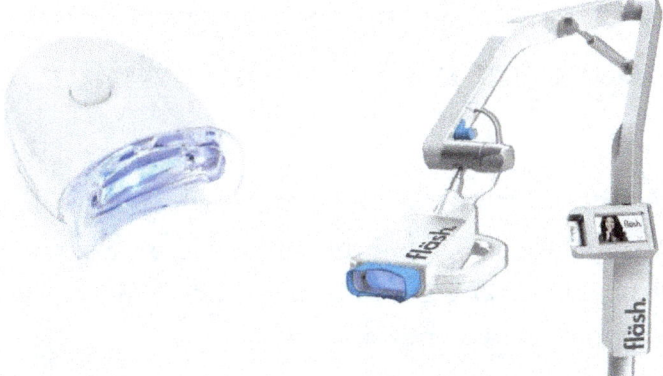

at-home LED light device   in-office LED light device

Always remember that in-office LED teeth whitening offers better results than the at-home version. That's because the professional LED devices dentists use are more powerful than any LED light that can be purchased over the counter.

Moreover, as in the case of teeth whitening trays, the gel used by your dentist will usually contain a higher amount of active ingredient, making the whitening process more effective.

At-home LED teeth whitening kits usually produce reasonably good results. However, the whitening you see is mainly the result of the gel and only in a smaller amount of the LED light.

How long does LED teeth whitening take to work?

After using an at-home kit, it can take up to 14 days to see the first whitening results. By contrast, in-office LED teeth whitening will get you faster results; it generally takes 1 to 3 appointments before you notice the first effects.

What should you look for when purchasing an LED teeth whitening kit?

The amount of active ingredient in the whitening gel determines how effective the bleaching treatment will be. So, you may want to choose a whitening gel with the highest amount of hydrogen peroxide or carbamide peroxide.

It is important to point out that some at-home whitening kits may contain a whitening agent that isn't exactly as strong as claimed.

The downside of choosing a gel with high amounts of active ingredients is that it increases the risk of tooth sensitivity after the treatment. As a result, discussing the options with your dentist will help you choose a product that is best suited for your dental health.

Additionally, reading the product reviews is another way to find answers to many questions you may have, such as:

- How effective is the product?
- Does the treatment create any discomfort?
- Does the LED light create any adverse side effects?
- How long does the treatment take?
- How effective is it in the long term?

LED teeth whitening pros

- At-home LED teeth whitening is reasonably effective even though the LED light doesn't add much value.
- The price is affordable compared to the in-office method.
- An interesting fact observed is that the LED light (even if it doesn't add much therapeutic value) helps people stick to their whitening routines, which is a crucial element. It may be a psychological thing that happens when patients have to use the gel plus the blue or indigo light.

Risks and drawbacks

As with most teeth whitening procedures, teeth sensitivity or gum discomfort are side effects that may appear during the treatment. Usually, these symptoms are mild and disappear relatively quickly. If the symptoms are severe and persistent, stop using the gel and consult your dentist.

These side effects generally appear when the whitening gels contain a higher amount of active ingredient.

On the other hand, Jerry Friedman, DDS, warns that if the LED lights are misused, adverse side effects may occur.

"If used incorrectly, it's possible to experience adverse side effects from using whitening gel with LED lights. Instead, I suggest they use whitening gels on their own or opt for a different over-the-counter whitening option," Dr. Friedman explains.

Zev Shulhof, DMD, MD, rarely recommends that his patients use LED lights at home because, in his opinion, the risk of tissue damage inside the mouth (from improper use) is too high to be worth quicker whitening results.

How to use LED teeth whitening?

Before using the whitening kit, read the product's instructions carefully. Each type of LED whitening can be slightly different, so make sure you follow the exact instructions.

TEETH WHITENING AT HOME
THE 6 BEST PRODUCTS EXPLORED AND COMPARED

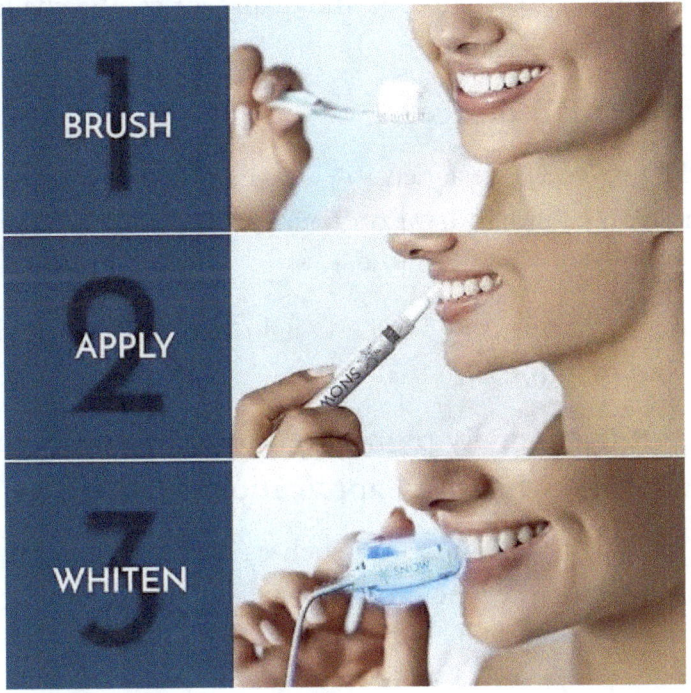

1. Brush and dry your teeth

Brush your teeth, then dry them by wiping with a tissue or your finger. Drying your teeth ensures the chemical agent adheres to your teeth better for enhanced whitening.

2. Apply the whitening gel

Some kits use an application pen to apply the serum to your teeth. One to two clicks of hydrogen peroxide gel is usually enough to whiten up to four teeth.

Other kits use a device tray to hold the gel on your teeth, similar to the whitening tray method. The downside of this method is that most whitening kits offer only one size to accommodate the wide range of mouths that will be using the device.

If the fitting isn't quite proper, the treatment can be challenging. Using an in-office custom-made tray may be a better solution.

3. Use the LED device

The LED device is designed to enhance the whitening process. Use the blue or indigo light on your teeth as directed (generally around 10 minutes). Do not overuse.

Remember that misusing the LED light can cause tissue damage inside your mouth.

4. Do not use heavily pigmented food or drinks for one hour after the whitening application

Avoid staining foods or drinks such as coffee, red wine, or tea at least one hour after the procedure.

How long does a treatment with LED light last?

Like the whitening tray method, an LED teeth whitening procedure may last 6 months or even up to one year if you practice good oral hygiene and maintenance measures.

Best products: LED Light Whitening

- Crest Whitening Emulsions Leave-on Teeth Whitening Gel Kit With LED Accelerator Light

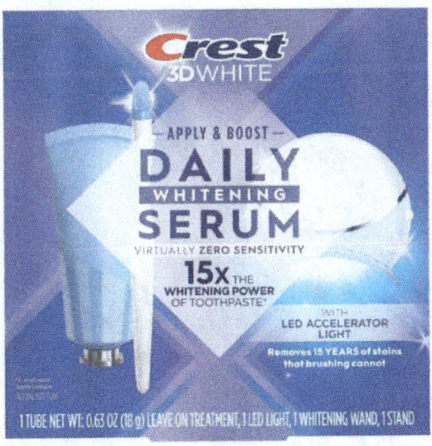

George Ghidrai, MD: "I tested Crest Whitening Emulsions with LED Light on 10 of my patients. 6 of them had very good results, 3 reported temporary teeth sensitivity but were satisfied with the outcome, and one could not use the LED Light. All in all, positive results."

- Auraglow Teeth Whitening Kit

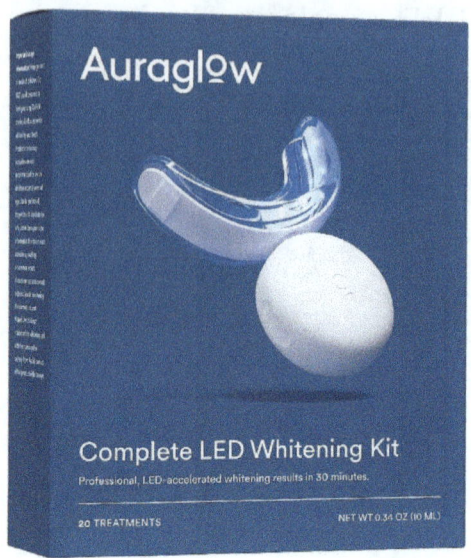

Product Description: "The complete LED teeth whitening kit uses our dental-grade teeth whitening formula with the power of LED light to deliver whiter teeth faster. Our 35% carbamide peroxide gel has been clinically proven to remove stains, and our advanced LED light is one of the most powerful at-home accelerators on the market."

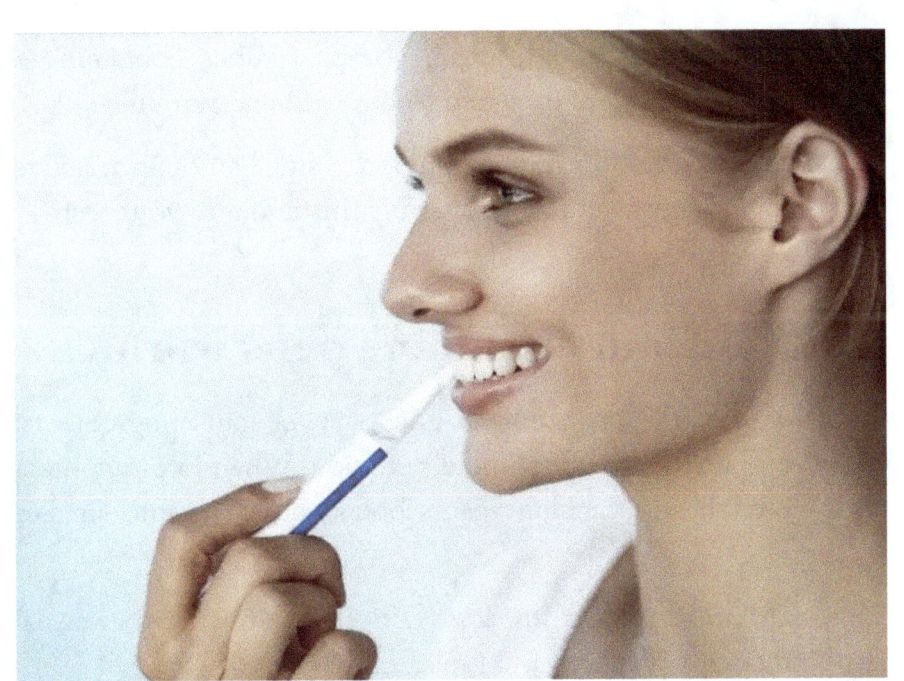

7. Teeth Whitening Pens

Teeth whitening pens are small, compact tubes containing a whitening gel. They are designed to be small and portable.

When you twist the bottom of the pen, a small amount of active gel seeps into a brush. You then apply this liquid to your teeth.

How do teeth whitening pens work?

Teeth whitening pens contain one of two active ingredients: hydrogen peroxide or carbamide peroxide. When left in contact with teeth, these bleaching agents break the stains into smaller pieces.

This will make the stains less concentrated, and the visual appearance of your teeth will look brighter.

What to expect from teeth whitening pens?

Teeth whitening pens are ideal for minor touch-ups to your teeth's whiteness. They give excellent results in combination with other teeth whitening procedures, especially with professional methods.

Eric Chengyu Xu, DDS from Precision Dentistry of Olympia, recommends whitening pens to his patients for speedy touch-ups and as an adjunct to a more rigorous whitening regimen. "If you are going to use a whitening pen, use it for touch-ups, not as the main context of your whitening life," points out Dr. Xu.

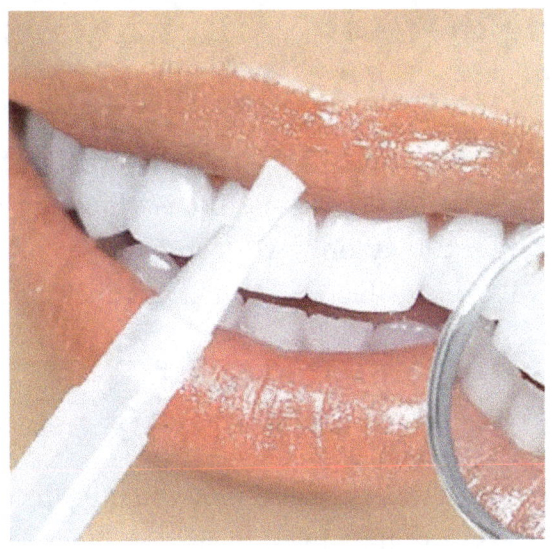

Teeth whitening pens work best on minor stains; they will more likely whiten yellow stains but have little effect on brown or gray stains.

"The whitening result will not last very long, and it is unlikely they will produce dramatic color changes in your teeth," mentions Zev Shulhof DMD, MD.

Ideally, you will use teeth whitening pens as a temporary solution prior to a special event or meeting to add a last-minute touch-up to your teeth whiteness.

Craig Barney, DMD, from Kennewick Dental, explains: "If I had to compare their potency, I'd rank them below professional treatments and most other at-home treatments, such as whitening strips, that I've also tried. But I still think they're a good option to have on hand (or in the purse)."

How long do teeth whitening pens take to work?

It takes only a few seconds to use them and about 30 minutes for them to do their work. While their whitening effect won't last indefinitely, and they only work in cases of minor staining, this method will give visible results in a relatively short time.

What should you look for when purchasing teeth whitening pens?

According to a 2016 study, there is no significant difference in the effectiveness of the two bleaching agents, so a pen containing either hydrogen peroxide or carbamide peroxide should be a good option.

When you look for whitening pens, check the amount of active ingredients each contains. Pens with a higher concentration of bleaching agent tend to give better whitening results. Teeth whitening pens typically contain between 6 and 9 percent hydrogen peroxide.

A higher concentration of active ingredients may also mean a higher risk of teeth sensitivity after the treatment. However, because teeth whitening pens contain relatively lower amounts of bleaching agents, teeth sensitivity, if it does appear, is usually mild and temporary.

As with other bleaching products, it is always important to discuss your options with your dentist and check customer reviews.

Dr. Jerry Friedman, North Jersey Oral & Maxillofacial Surgery, warns that you need to be careful when selecting a whitening pen: "Teeth whitening pens can be pretty effective, but not all are created equally. Reputable brands are worth investing in if you want results you can count on," Dr. Friedman believes.

Teeth whitening pens pros

Eric Chengyu Xu, DDS, states that whitening pens "could be called the simplest of the at-home whitening treatment options, and they are also the most portable."

Here are whitening pens' most important benefits:

- **Convenience** is one of the main benefits of teeth whitening pens. They are small and compact and can easily fit in your pocket or purse so you can take them anywhere for quick applications.

- **Easy to use.** While instructions may vary from product to product, the application mainly involves a few seconds of twisting and applying. You will use a small brush applicator to apply the solution directly to your teeth.

- **Cost.** Teeth whitening pens are some of the most affordable teeth whitening products on the market.

- **Flexibility.** Unlike whitening strips or trays, whitening pens can be used to target specific teeth (even a single tooth) in your mouth.

Risks and drawbacks

- Teeth whitening pens are temporary solutions, and the whitening results will not last long.

- They work best with minor stains and have little effect in case of more severe staining.

- Side effects such as teeth sensitivity or gum irritation may appear. However, these symptoms are usually mild and temporary.

Moreover, Dr. Jerry Friedman suggests that "pens are generally better for those with sensitive teeth because they are more gentle to use."

How to use teeth whitening pens?

Whitening pens are very easy to use. While instructions may vary from product to product, the application mainly involves four steps.

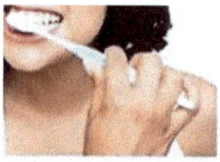

1. Brush and dry your teeth

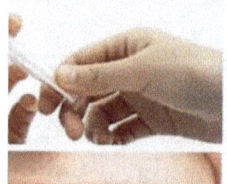

2. Prepare the whitening pen

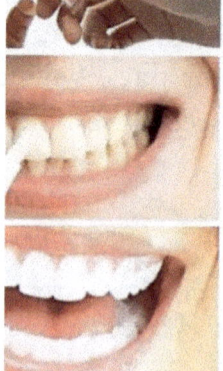

3. Apply the gel

4. Do not eat or rinse for 30 minutes

1. Brush and dry your teeth

Bush your teeth with a soft-bristle toothbrush, then dry them by wiping with a tissue or your finger.

2. Prepare the whitening pen

Remove the top cap of the pen and twist the bottom until you see the gel on the brush tip.

3. Apply the gel

Apply a thin layer of whitening gel to each tooth's surface, ensuring the entire surface is in contact with the gel.

4. Do not eat or rinse

Avoid eating, rinsing, and drinking for at least 30 minutes after applying the product. It needs to stay in contact with your teeth to be effective. Rinsing or drinking can wash it away, minimizing the whitening effects.

You can use whitening pens twice daily, but this is not a general rule. Eric Chengyu Xu, DDS, indicates that whitening pens "are not meant to be used like other at-home whitening treatments that you use every day or nearly every day for several weeks to yield maximum results."

How long does a treatment with teeth whitening pens last?

Zev Shulhof, DMD, MD, explains that whitening pens are best used "as a maintenance option for between professional whitening treatments rather than as a treatment on their own."

A treatment with whitening pens does not last for too long. "A few days to a week is a reasonable approximation," Craig Barney, DMD, believes.

As mentioned, teeth whitening pens are ideal for minor touch-ups to your teeth's whiteness. For example, you can benefit from these touch-ups before an important event; the results will last until the event ends.

Best products: Whitening Pens

- Auraglow Whitening Pen

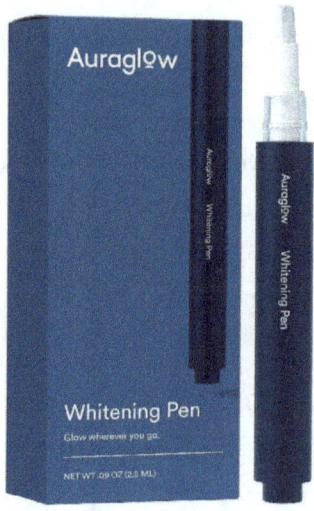

Craig Barney DMD: "The top teeth-whitening pen on the market is the AuraGlow Whitening Pen. It boasts a high concentration of whitening agents, delivers steady and reliable results, and is user-friendly to boot."

Eric Chengyu Xu, DDS: "AuraGlow Teeth Whitening Pen is the top option for whitening teeth with a pen. It's effective and easy to use. Given its results and our experience with it, we can recommend it without reservation."

- Colgate Optic White Overnight Teeth Whitening Pen

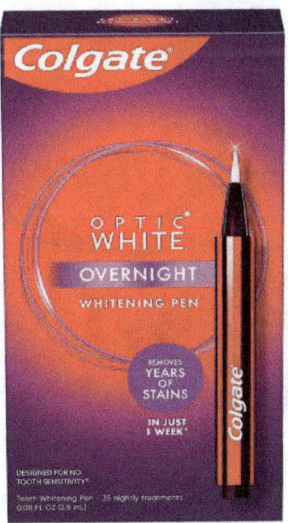

George Ghidrai, MD: "The Colgate Optic Whitening Pen provides surprisingly good results. It can be used as described - with the gel left over the night - but also for minor touch-ups during the day."

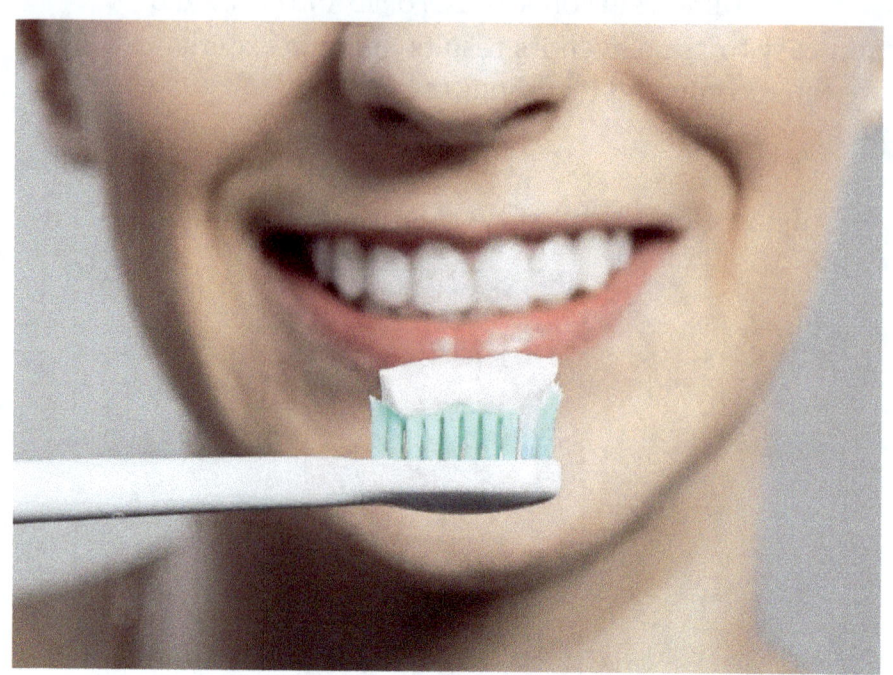

8. Teeth whitening toothpaste

A whitening toothpaste is an effective way to remove surface stains from the teeth, but it cannot change the color of your teeth.

Regularly using these types of toothpaste can help maintain teeth's natural color by removing daily surface stains and avoiding major darkening.

Craig Barney, DMD from Kennewick Dental, summarizes the effectiveness of whitening toothpaste: **"Based on my experience, whitening toothpaste can somewhat assist in eliminating surface stains and preventing the formation of new ones. It can sustain the effects of bleaching procedures but usually doesn't change the basic color of one's teeth."**

How does whitening toothpaste work?

A tooth whitening toothpaste contains various types of ingredients:

- Abrasives such as baking soda, hydrated silica, or charcoal
- Bleaching agents (e.g., hydrogen peroxide and carbamide peroxide)
- Fluoride, to prevent cavities and gum disease
- Potassium nitrate, to prevent tooth sensitivity caused by bleaching agents
- Other ingredients, such as colorants, surfactants, antiredeposition agents, etc.

The abrasives are the main ingredients in whitening toothpaste. They act on your teeth to rub away surface stains and polish them.

Whitening toothpaste only works on external stains (those that originate from external sources, such as drinks, foods, or tobacco products). It does not affect internal stains (stains that start inside the tooth, for example, from aging or internal decay).

Whitening toothpastes don't have a concentration of bleaching agents high enough to change the color of teeth, so the whitening effects are minimal.

In conclusion, whitening toothpaste offers minor stain removal that maintains your existing tooth color instead of whitening it to another shade.

What to expect from a whitening toothpaste?

If you are thinking of switching to whitening toothpaste, it is essential to start with realistic expectations.

When regularly used, whitening toothpastes may be effective on external stains, but they will not lighten the shade of your teeth nor affect the internal stains.

Eric Chengyu Xu, DDS from Precision Dentistry of Olympia, indicates that "**Whitening toothpaste works best as part of a regular oral hygiene routine to prevent and reduce stains.**"

Many patients who think these types of toothpaste will brighten their teeth tend to use it more often than directed, which can damage the tooth enamel.

If you want a more dramatic change, you should use whitening toothpaste **in combination** with other, more efficient bleaching procedures (such as professional whitening, whitening gels or strips).

Shahrooz Yazdani, DDS, CEO and Director of Yazdani Family Dentistry and Costello Family Dentistry, recommends the use of whitening toothpaste in two cases:

1. "We recommend teeth-whitening toothpaste for patients looking for a simple and cost-effective way to maintain their teeth's brightness and reduce minor discoloration."

2. "It is also a good option for patients who have completed professional whitening treatments and wish to prolong their results."

How long does whitening toothpaste take to work?

Whitening toothpastes are designed for regular, long-term use. As a result, you should not expect to see visible results in less than two weeks.

Craig Barney, DMD, stresses the importance of regular, long-term use: "To see any kind of result, you have to use the toothpaste devotedly as part of your routine - you can't just use it off and on and expect to see any change."

Moreover, "to achieve noticeable results, one should use a whitening toothpaste for no less than 2-4 weeks," continues Dr. Barney.

What should you look for when purchasing teeth whitening toothpaste?

First, make sure that you use a whitening toothpaste with the American Dental Association (ADA) seal. This seal shows that the toothpaste brand that uses it is safe and effective. Other countries may use similar types of seals.

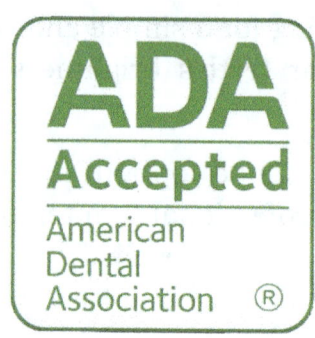

American Dental Association (ADA) seal

Ensure that the toothpaste contains active abrasive ingredients (such as baking soda, hydrated silica, or charcoal), as whitening toothpastes rely heavily on abrasives for their results.

Look for options that include fluoride and potassium nitrate, which are gentler on your teeth and help prevent tooth sensitivity caused by bleaching agents.

Scott Cardall, DMD, MS, suggests patients look for whitening toothpaste that also contains **stannous fluoride**:

"I prefer toothpastes that contain certain active ingredients like stannous fluoride, a type of fluoride with small amounts of tin that research has shown contributes additional benefits beyond the regular sodium fluoride," Dr. Cardall advises.

Teeth whitening toothpaste pros

"Whitening toothpaste has multiple benefits; it's what I call a 'two-for-one' product. Not only does it help to keep teeth nice and white, but it also contains the cavity-fighting ingredient fluoride," Eric Chengyu Xu, DDS, says.

Here are some of the main benefits:

- Very easy to use
- Lower in cost than other over-the-counter whitening products
- When regularly used, it can successfully remove minor stains
- Most of the time, it is safe to use

Dr. Zev Schulhof, Iconic Implants, states: "When it comes to at-home teeth whitening, the product I am most likely to recommend is whitening toothpaste. It is the easiest product to use and generally has the least amount of side effects."

Risks and drawbacks

If you overuse toothpaste, the abrasive ingredients can damage the enamel. Therefore, it is imperative to use whitening toothpaste as instructed (either by your dentist or by reading the product's instructions). Generally, you should not use whitening toothpaste more than twice daily.

Other side effects may include teeth sensitivity and gum irritation. However, these rarely occur with whitening toothpaste, especially when the toothpaste contains potassium nitrate or fluoride.

How to use whitening toothpaste?

First, following the package instructions or your dentist's recommendations is essential.

In general, you should use the same brushing technique as you usually do. Here is a short reminder on how to brush your teeth correctly.

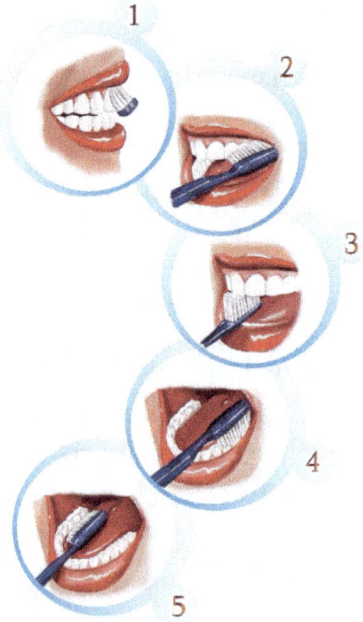

Make sure to follow these tips as well:

- Use a gentle touch when brushing
- Select a soft-bristled toothbrush
- Brush no more often than twice a day

- Limit brushing sessions to no longer than two minutes at a time

You may also want to limit the foods and drinks that stained your teeth in the first place (coffee, red wine, berries). If this is too challenging, don't forget to rinse your teeth with plenty of water after eating or drinking these types of foods.

You should also avoid smoking or using smokeless tobacco products to avoid the formation of brown stains.

How long does a treatment with whitening toothpaste last?

Shahrooz Yazdani, DDS, believes that "treatment with whitening toothpaste should be ongoing as part of your daily oral hygiene routine. Most whitening toothpastes are safe for long-term use and should be used twice daily, just like regular toothpaste." points out Dr. Yazdani.

You may see good results as long as you use the toothpaste regularly and as instructed. Avoid (or limit) staining foods and tobacco, and have realistic expectations.

Remember, teeth whitening toothpaste cannot whiten your teeth. It can be an effective way to remove surface stains from the teeth, but for better bleaching results, you may wish to combine this method with other, more effective bleaching procedures.

Best products: Whitening Toothpaste

- Colgate Optic White

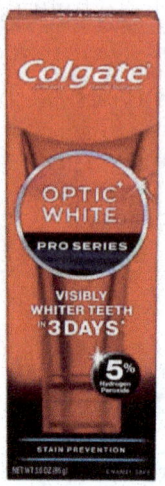
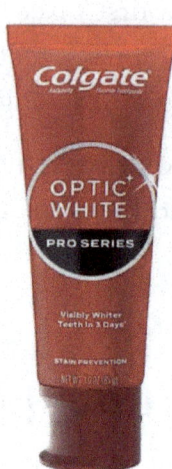

Craig Barney DMD: "To me, the best toothpaste for whitening is Colgate Optic White. The reason is simple: it has hydrogen peroxide as an ingredient, which helps remove stains — a little like using bleach (but safe for your mouth, of course). And in just two weeks, you're supposed to see a noticeably whiter smile, with continued improvement if you keep brushing."

Eric Chengyu Xu, DDS: "To my way of thinking, the best-performing toothpaste for whitening is Colgate Optic White. You have to use it for a while to get results. The main reason it works is that the first ingredient is hydrogen peroxide, which is also the active ingredient in most bleaching gels used by dentists."

- Crest Pro-Health

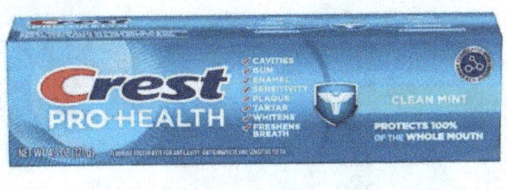

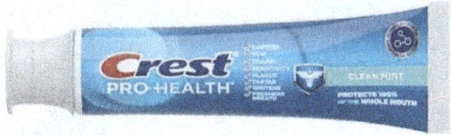

Scott Cardall, DMD, MS: "I prefer toothpastes that contain certain active ingredients like stannous fluoride, a type of fluoride with small amounts of tin that research has shown contributes additional benefits beyond the regular sodium fluoride. Whitening toothpaste that has stannous fluoride includes Crest-Pro Health, Sensodyne Rapid Relief, and others."

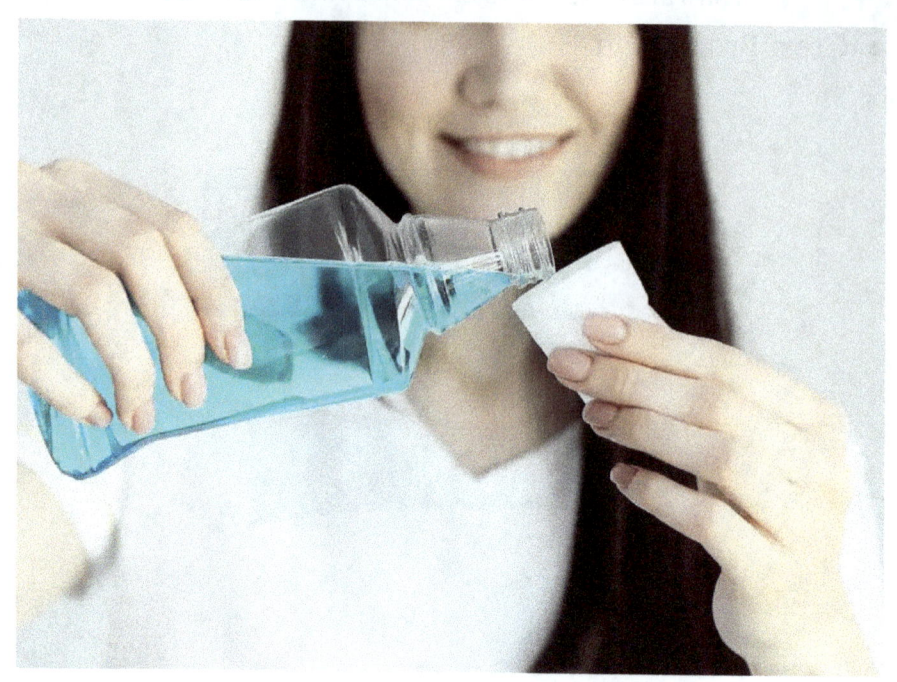

9. Teeth whitening rinses

Teeth whitening rinses are particular kinds of mouthwashes that typically contain hydrogen peroxide as the bleaching agent.

A teeth whitening rinse can help remove surface stains from the teeth and may help you lighten your teeth slightly.

Craig Barney, DMD, from Kennewick Dental, points out that a whitening mouthwash can be a "**safeguard against relapse, even though it cannot replace a full-strength treatment.**"

How do teeth whitening rinses work?

The bleaching agent contained in the mouthwash penetrates the surface of your teeth and breaks down the pigments responsible for tooth staining. This will work better on external stains, which have built up because of lifestyle factors like coffee, tea, red wine, or tobacco.

Dr. Zev Schulhof, Iconic Implants, believes that "whitening mouthwashes are moderately effective at removing surface stains and helping teeth look whiter but aren't effective enough to produce dramatic results on their own."

What to expect from teeth whitening rinses?

Generally, whitening mouthwashes contain a low concentration of bleaching agent (around 2%). As a result, a whitening rinse will only be able to lighten your teeth slightly. Moreover, these products work best for minor staining and have little or no effect on significant discolorations or prominent staining.

Nevertheless, whitening mouthwashes work very well **when combined** with other at-home and professional teeth whitening treatments.

Jasveen Singh, DMD, Pediatric Dentist and the Owner of Pediatric Dentistry And Beyond in Boston, stresses this fact: "While whitening mouthwashes can slightly improve the brightness of your teeth, their real power shines through when used in combination with other methods."

Craig Barney, DMD, is convinced that "results from a potent means of whitening, like professional applications or the use of strips or gels, can be maintained by employing mouthwash."

"That means that altogether, these different products used for different times of the day add up to better oral health, better retained and longer lasting whitening effects, and make your mouth more attractive," Dr. Barney explains.

How long does a whitening mouthwash take to work?

For a whitening mouthwash to be effective, you need to make it a consistent part of your oral care routine. It is usually recommended that you use the whitening rinse twice daily.

Even if you use the mouthwash according to the instructions, you must wait at least a month for the first results. For a more effective procedure, try combining the whitening rinse with other teeth whitening treatments.

What should you look for when purchasing whitening mouthwash?

A good teeth whitening mouthwash will include ingredients that do more than whiten your teeth. "Whitening mouthwashes are fantastic for maintaining the whiteness achieved through more impressive treatments and play a dual part by keeping your breath fresh and reducing plaque and bacteria," Jasveen Singh, DMD, points out.

As a result, when you choose a whitening mouthwash, look for these types of ingredients:

- The bleaching agent: most of the time, a 2% concentration of hydrogen peroxide.

- Look for added anti-plaque and anti-tartar ingredients like *cetylpyridinium* chloride or *pyrophosphates*. A mouthwash that prevents plaque and tartar from building up goes a long way toward a brighter and healthier smile.

- Fluoride keeps your enamel strong and healthy and reduces tooth sensitivity.

Look for an alcohol-free mouthwash, as alcohol can dry out your mouth and worsen symptoms of dry mouth (xerostomia). Dry mouth is a condition which affects the flow of saliva, causing your mouth to feel dry and uncomfortable.

Avoid mouthwashes that are dark in color, as the color can actually stain your teeth.

Finally, ensure the mouthwash has been approved by the American Dental Association (ADA) or similar organizations worldwide.

Teeth whitening rinses pros

- easy to use and will only take around 2 minutes of your time every day
- reasonable price

- because the bleaching agent has a low concentration, whitening rinses are a safe teeth whitening option

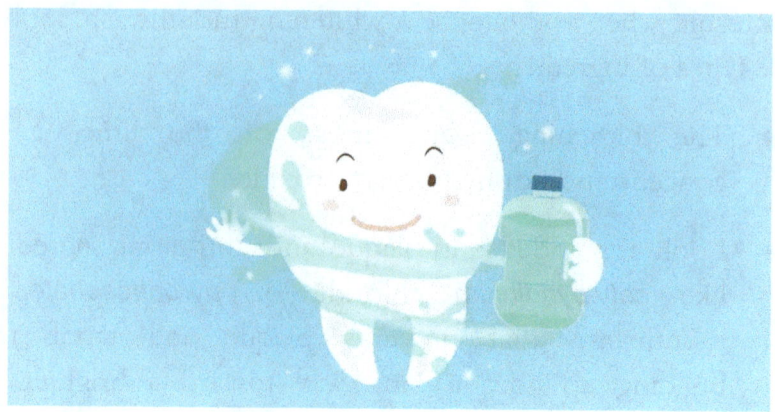

Risks and drawbacks

The amounts contained in a whitening mouthwash are considered safe and will not harm your enamel. Teeth sensitivity and gum irritation are rare side effects of over-the-counter whitening rinses.

If the mouthwash contains alcohol, it may dry your mouth. If you suffer from dry mouth (xerostomia), your symptoms may worsen. Therefore, try to look for an alcohol-free mouthwash.

How to use teeth whitening rinses?

You will most often use an over-the-counter product. Over-the-counter mouthwashes contain a limited amount of bleaching agent (usually 2%).

However, it is also possible to use a mouthwash prescribed by your dentist. A whitening mouthwash prescribed by your dentist will contain more hydrogen peroxide. It may also include therapeutic ingredients for other oral health concerns (such as gum disease) and ingredients to prevent tooth sensitivity.

Always follow the recommended usage instructions for whitening mouthwashes.

Using teeth rinses is easy and straightforward. Most products require you to swish the solution around your mouth for 60 seconds twice daily. Remember not to swallow!

Dr. Jerry Friedman, North Jersey Oral & Maxillofacial Surgery, adds another piece of advice: "With a whitening mouthwash, the key for maximum effectiveness is to avoid rinsing your mouth out with water afterward, as well as avoiding eating or drinking for 10-30 minutes afterward."

Another essential aspect is that you should be committed to using it in the long term.

How long does a treatment with whitening mouthwash last?

For a whitening mouthwash to be effective, you need to use it in the long term.

We have asked Eric Chengyu Xu, DDS from Precision Dentistry of Olympia, how long he recommends his patients use whitening rinses. Dr. Xu had a definite answer:

"I suggest to my patients that they use whitening mouth rinses in a very specific way if they want to get the best results. First, I tell them to use the rinse twice a day—once in the morning and once in the evening—for a minimum duration of 3 months. Second, I instruct them to use the mouth rinse not as a quick swish and spit but as a 60-second rinse-and-hold. I tell them that the holding part is just as important to the effectiveness of the product as the swishing part."

Your dentist or dental hygienist can tell you how long you should use it. They can also determine if you are a good candidate for other whitening treatments and recommend the best techniques for your situation.

Best products: Whitening Rinses

- Crest 3D White Brilliance Whitening Mouthwash, Alcohol Free

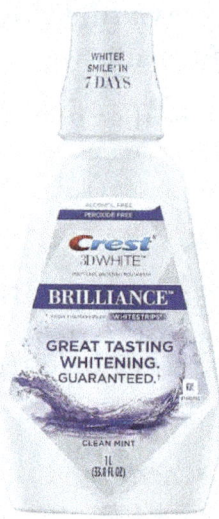

Craig Barney DMD: "To me, Crest 3D White Brilliance Whitening Mouthwash seems to be the best mouthwash for whitening teeth that one can find. I think of this because I've tried it a few times and was satisfied with it. After rinsing, my teeth whitened a little and were left clean and fresh."

Eric Chengyu Xu, DDS: "From my perspective, Crest 3D White Brilliance is the finest mouthwash available for teeth whitening. It works well and doesn't require you to do anything out of the norm. Just swish and spit like you would with any other mouthwash, and rinse with water afterward."

- Listerine Advanced White

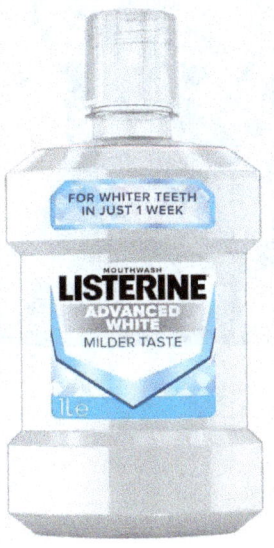

Jasveen Singh, DMD: " I'm a big fan of Listerine White Anticavity Fluoride Mouthwash. It contains hydrogen peroxide, which is great for lifting surface stains and brightening your smile, and fluoride, which boosts enamel strength and fights off cavities. Most people I know really like the taste and hardly ever have any issues with sensitivity."

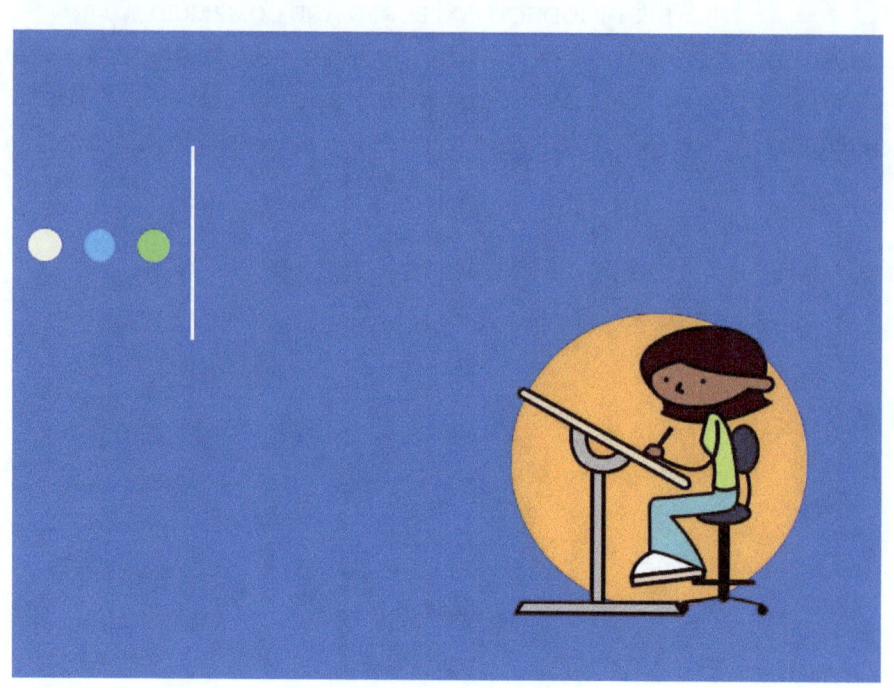

10. Conclusions

At-home teeth whitening is less expensive than in-office whitening treatments but can achieve excellent results with patients who use them consistently and for sufficient time.

This book has thoroughly examined and compared the 6 best-known at-home teeth whitening methods.

Let's explore some key takeaways:

1. **Talk to your dentist before using any over-the-counter whitening products.**

   This essential step can save you time, effort, and money.

   Your dentist will help you pick an efficient product best suited for your dental health. He will also explain how to use it correctly and ensure that the side effects are kept to a minimum.

2. **Most of the time, you will have to use more than a single product for optimum results.**

   For example, results from an efficient whitening procedure (such as whitening trays or strips, or professional bleaching) can be maintained (or even enhanced) by regularly using whitening toothpaste and rinses.

   Whitening pens are excellent for quick touch-ups but are best used in combination with other bleaching treatments.

3. **Most experts regard custom-made trays with professional whitening gels as the preferred at-home treatment.**

Scott Cardall, DMD, MS: "I recommend custom-fitted whitening trays with professional-grade whitening gels to be worn at home. This ensures better contact between the whitening agent and teeth, leading to more consistent whitening results."

Shahrooz Yazdani, DDS: "We like to use at-home kits, which involve using custom trays that you wear over your teeth each day to achieve results over a more extended period. These trays contain peroxide gels, and the custom-fit trays allow maximum contact with the gel to achieve optimal results at home."

4. **Whitening pens are considered excellent for quick touch-ups** and are best used in combination with other bleaching treatments.

5. **Whitening strips have two main advantages**: they are very easy to use and affordable. On the downside, they also carry a higher risk of side effects, such as tooth sensitivity or gum irritation.

6. **Whitening toothpaste is the product with the least amount of side effects**. Together with **whitening rinses**, it can effectively improve the look of mild surface staining while maintaining the results of other whitening treatments.

Jerry Friedman, DDS, likes to recommend a combination of whitening toothpaste and whitening mouthwash to his patients. "This combination can effectively improve the look of mild surface staining without causing issues such as increased sensitivity, which we sometimes see with treatments such as whitening strips or gels. Whitening toothpaste is also one of the easiest options to work into your dental routine, so patients are more likely to stick with them," he explains.

Dr. Zev Schulhof, Iconic Implants, also recommends whitening toothpaste: "When it comes to at-home teeth whitening, the product I am most likely to recommend is whitening toothpaste. It is the easiest product to use and generally has the least amount of side effects. Plus, many patients who really want to achieve whiter teeth are even more motivated to keep up with brushing at least twice daily if they are using a whitening toothpaste."

Our experts

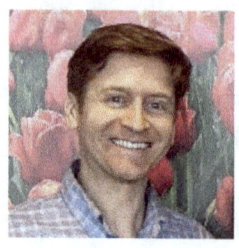

Scott Cardall, DMD, MS

Scott Cardall, DMD, MS, Owner Orthodontist at Orem Orthodontics, was born and raised in Laguna Hills, California, 10 minutes from the beach and 20 minutes from Disneyland. After graduating as a co-valedictorian from Brigham Young University, Dr. Cardall attended the Harvard School of Dental Medicine. There, he received the highest score in his class and the country on the important part one board exam, as well as became a published primary author of a scientific study on remote learning which has been cited more than 50 times in the scientific literature.

Dr. Cardall then completed his residency back on the West Coast at Oregon Health & Science University in Portland, Oregon. He received his Specialty Certificate in Orthodontics and a Masters in Science with a thesis on digital models.

"We, orthodontists, get asked about teeth whitening a lot, as we are often the first dental provider patients think about when they consider the aesthetics of their teeth; often, the first time a patient thinks about whitening their teeth is when they are straightening their teeth," explains Dr. Cardall.

TEETH WHITENING AT HOME
THE 6 BEST PRODUCTS EXPLORED AND COMPARED

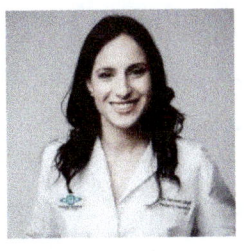

Jasveen Singh, DMD

Dr. Jasveen Singh is a Pediatric Dentist and the Owner of Pediatric Dentistry And Beyond in Boston.
She is a dedicated and compassionate pediatric dentist serving the community of Tewksbury and beyond. Dr. Singh's journey in the field of dentistry began in Canton, MA, where she nurtured her passion for oral health. Her educational path led her to Tufts University School of Dental Medicine, where she graduated in 2015. Following a year of experience as a general dentist, her unwavering dedication to pediatric dentistry led her to Boston University, where she pursued specialized training for two years to become a renowned expert in her field.

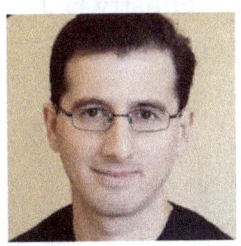

Shahrooz Yazdani, DDS

Dr. Shahrooz Yazdani is the CEO & Director at Costello Family Dentistry.
After earning his DDS degree with Honours from the University of Toronto in 1998, Dr. Yazdani completed a 2-year general practice residency in North Carolina. Residencies like this are optional; in fact, less than 1% of general dentists choose

to pursue this sort of residency.

Dr. Yazdani's commitment to his trade didn't stop there. He then completed over 1,000 hours of comprehensive continuing education offered by the Kois Center, as well as a 330-hour implant and bone grafting course through Ti-Max in Toronto. In 2001, he opened Yazdani Dental and brought his many years of experience to clients in both Kanata and Kemptville. Dr. Yazdani believes strongly in helping others, and enjoys his work immensely.

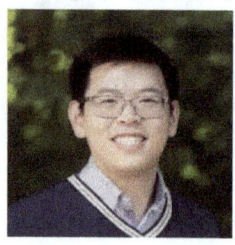

Eric Xu, DDS

Dr. Eric Xu, DDS, from Precision Dentistry of Olympia, has a passion for transforming smiles and improving oral health. With his comprehensive training in general and family dentistry, with a special focus on restorative dentistry, implant, and cosmetic dentistry, Dr. Xu brings a wealth of evidence-based expertise and a commitment to excellence to his practice.

Dr. Xu's academic journey began at the University of Washington, where he graduated cum laude in 2018 with a B.Sc. in Biochemistry and a minor in Bioethics. His exceptional academic performance and rigorous scientific education showcased his commitment to a solid foundation in the field. Driven by his thirst for knowledge and pursuit of dental excellence, he excelled at the esteemed University of Washington School of Dentistry, graduating at the top of his class, and earning his DDS with distinction in 2023.

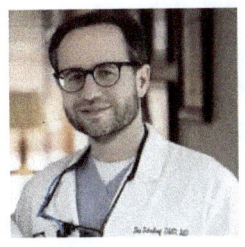

Zev Schulhof, DMD, MD

Dr. Zev Schulhof, Iconic Implants, is an oral and maxillofacial surgeon as well as a physician, and attending surgeon at Mount Sinai Hospital in New York City. Dr. Schulhof received his undergraduate degree in Judaic studies from Touro College in New York City and his dental degree from the University of Medicine and Dentistry of New Jersey (now Rutgers). He attended medical school at Mount Sinai School of Medicine, graduating in 2003. He completed his six-year oral and maxillofacial surgery residency at Mount Sinai Medical Center in New York, where he was Chief Resident from 2005 to 2006. Dr. Schulhof is a Diplomate of the American Board of Oral & Maxillofacial Surgery as well as a Member of the American Association of Oral & Maxillofacial Surgeons, and the International Association of Oral & Maxillofacial Surgeons. He is also the current President of the American Academy of Facial Cosmetics.

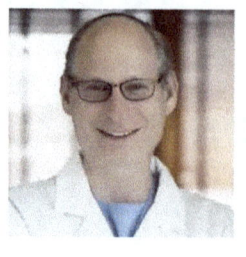

Jerry Friedman, DDS

Dr. Jerry Friedman, DDS, from North Jersey Oral & Maxillofacial Surgery, received his undergraduate degree in pre-med and Judaic studies from Touro College in New York City and his dental degree from Columbia University School of Dentistry in New York City. He completed a General Practice Dental Residency at Beth Israel Hospital and his Oral Surgery Residency at Mount Sinai Medical Center in New York City. Dr. Friedman has professional affiliations with the International Congress of Oral Implantologists and the American Association of Oral and Maxillofacial Surgeons. He is a Diplomate of the American Board of Oral and Maxillofacial Surgery and the American Dental Society of Anesthesiology.

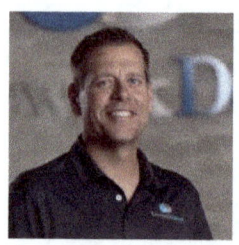

Craig Barney, DMD

Dr. Barney received his Doctor of Dental Medicine (DMD) at Case Western Reserve University in Cleveland, OH, in 2005. Prior to dental school, he earned his Bachelor's degree in Zoology from Brigham Young University.

Dr. Barney has been practicing dentistry since 2005. In 2008, he took over "Taylor-Made Smiles" from Dr. James Taylor, DDS. Since then, Dr. Barney has strived to continue improving technology, materials, and techniques so that we can offer the best care possible to our patients.

References

Medical News Today: *What to know about teeth whitening strips*

Belmont Dental: *Do Teeth Whitening Strips Work?*

Health Line: *Do Teeth Whitening Strips Work?*

Colgate: *White Strips for Teeth Whitening: Do They Really Work and How to Use Them Effectively*

Colgate: *How Custom Whitening Trays Brighten Your Smile*

Dental Studio: *How To Use Take-Home Teeth Whitening Trays from Your Dentist*

Miami Perfect Smile: *Tooth whitening tray: Everything you need to know*

Crest: *Teeth Whitening Trays: How they Work and Alternatives*

Colgate: *How Does LED Teeth Whitening Work?*

JS Dental Lab: *LED Whitening: Is it a gimmick?*

The Strategist: *Do At-Home LED Teeth Whiteners Actually Work?*

Colgate: *Teeth Whitening Pens 101*

Crest: *How Does a Teeth Whitening Pen Work?*

Landmark Dental Care: *Cosmetic Dentistry Questions: At Home Teeth Whitening Pens – How do They Work?*

Byte: *Do Teeth Whitening Pens Actually Work?*

The Dental District: *Benefits and Disadvantages of Teeth-Whitening Pen*

Matthews Family Dentistry: *Teeth Whitening Toothpaste: Do They Really Work?*

123 Dentist: *How Effective Are Whitening Toothpastes?*

Health: *Is Whitening Toothpaste Bad for Your Teeth?*

Colgate: *Teeth Whitening Toothpaste: Does It Work?*

Colgate: *The Best Mouthwash for Teeth Whitening: What to Look For*

Westside Family Dentistry: *Effective Ways to Whiten Your Teeth*

Lane & Associates Family Dentistry: *Can Mouthwash Help Whiten Teeth?*

About the Author

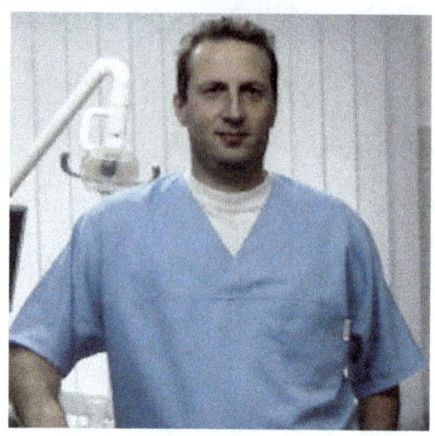

George Ghidrai MD

George Ghidrai, MD, is a General Dental Practitioner with over 20 years of experience. As a dental practitioner, Dr. Ghidrai has been actively treating patients at three dental clinics over the past 20 years.

Dr. Ghidrai's primary areas of expertise include cosmetic dentistry, tooth restoration, and prosthetic dentistry. In addition to being involved in direct patient care, he has also devoted much of his time to patient education. In 2013, he created *Infodentis.com*, a website that provides patients with extensive information on various dental procedures and mouth conditions.

Expertise

- Teeth Whitening and Cosmetic Dentistry
- Prosthetic and Implant Dentistry
- General Dentistry
- Content Writing

Education

Dr. George Ghidrai obtained his bachelor's degree in dentistry from the University of Medicine and Pharmacy "Iuliu Hatieganu" in Cluj-Napoca, Romania. He then received his MD, specializing in "General Dentistry", at the same University in 2003.
He worked for three different dental clinics, spending time on a variety of clinical cases. At present, he owns a Dental Practice in his hometown, Clu-Napoca.

Experience

In addition to his clinical experience, Dr. Ghidrai has been actively involved in developing and creating patient-education content for his website *Infodentis.com* as well as for other websites and publications.

Books By This Author

Dental Implants:

The Complete Patient's Guide

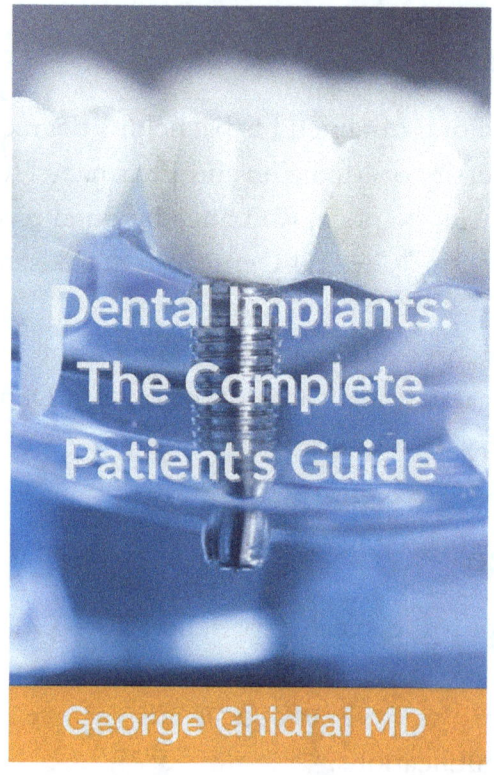